T0231480

Lymphoma
IN DOGS AND CATS

Wallace B. Morrison, *DVM, MS*

Diplomate ACVIM
(Small Animal Internal Medicine)

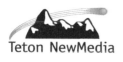

Teton NewMedia

Jackson, Wyoming
www.veterinarywire.com

Executive Editor: Carroll C. Cann
Development Editor: Susan L. Hunsberger
Creative Director: Sue Haun 5640 Design www.fiftysixforty.com
Production Manager: Mike Albiniak 5640 Design www.fiftysixforty.com

TetonNew Media
P.O. Box 4833
4125 South Hwy 89, Suite 1
Jackson, WY 83001

1-888-770-3165
veterinarywire.com
tetonnewmedia.com

Printed in the United States

ISBN# 1-893441-92-X

Print Number 5 4 3 2 1

Library of Congress Cataloging-in-Publication Data
Morrison, Wallace B.
        Lymphoma in dogs and cats / Wallace B. Morrison.
            p. cm.
        Includes bibliographical references (p.   ).
        ISBN 1-893441-92-X
        1. Dogs--Diseases. 2. Cats--Diseases. 3. Lymphomas in animals. I. Title.
        SF992.L94M67 2004
        636.7'089699'466--dc22

Dedication

This book is humbly dedicated to my fellow lunatics who graduated from Colorado State University, College of Veterinary and Biomedical Sciences on June 1, 1973. It was a glorious day. The weather was perfect, our parents and families were gathered around us in celebration, and we were young, full of high spirits, and eager to be veterinarians.

Colorado State University
DVM Class of 1973

Joseph W. Alexander, Jr.
Robert R. Anderson
Brian Baker
C. Ben Baker
Richard Beck
Steven R. Beyer*
Stephen Blake, Jr.
Christopher J. Boland
Richard A. Bowen
Hollis W. Brown*
Roger W. Chase
Donald D. Coates
Robert A. Cocanour
James Cook
Norman L. Defanti*
John F. Doherty, Jr.
Frederick M. Emerich
Boyd Emond
Lloyd Emond
Simon Escalada
William Fanning
Joel Folk
William Fredregill
Terry Gee
James P. Gibson*
Tom Gore
William W. Gould
Donald D. Hamilton

Ann M. Hargis
Donna L. Harper
Paul T. Hartman, Jr.
John C. Heideman
Dale R. Hill
Richard L. Hoffman, Jr.
Todd Humphreys
Drew Hutchinson
James R. Jackson
C. Dan Jones
Craig S. Kelly
Philip S. Kennedy
H. Craig Kiner
James I. Klopfenstein
Roger A. Kodel
Charles J. Koenig
Robert L. Kritsberg
William L. Lawrence
Linda A. Leadbetter
Martin R. Lee
Larry L. McMillan
Franklin D. Merritt*
Donald E. Moore
Wallace B. Morrison
William Musslewhite, Jr
David E. Nein
Thomas Noffsinger
William H. Patlogar

Thomas W. Pearson
R. Max Peterson
Leon Pielstick
Terrance L. Plog
Leon J. Pommer
Janis Potter–Bell
Gailyn D. Rodgers
Richard L. Rogers
Steve O. Sallen
Norman Schmeeckle
Delwin L. Seeba
Joe Shackelford*
Harvey Shaffer
Ronald E. Skinner
Dennis F. Smith
Michael A. Stewart
Gregg L. Voigt
Phillip J. Volkman
John V. White
William R. Williams
Gary L. Wood
James S. Young
David Youngs*

*Deceased

Dedication

Acknowledgements

I want to express my appreciation to several individuals who have contributed to making this book better than it would have otherwise been. Thanks to Dr. Kevin A. Hahn, Gulf Coast Veterinary Specialists, Houston, Texas for contributing specific content ideas for this book during two enjoyable dinners. I especially wish to thank Dr. Ted Valli from the University of Illinois and Dr. Rose Raskin of Purdue University for generously contributing many of the images contained in this book. Dr. Valli was also kind enough to write the figure legends for his images. Ted, Rose and Kevin are generous and gracious friends and colleagues who have made enormous contributions to our profession.

Preface

It seems to me that the field of oncology has advanced like no other in veterinary medicine. I believe that this advancement is the result of sharply focused dedication by many gifted clinicians, researchers, residents, graduate students, and pet owners, who together, make common cause against cancer. I believe that this progress owes much to the compelling nature of cancer. Cancer, like modern day terrorism, threatens us in a highly personal way. Cancer is an enemy that seems random in its targeting, and we must always assume it to be dangerous until proven benign and/or successfully overcome. Like modern terrorism, cancer seems totally indifferent to the sadness, pain, and suffering that it can visit on healthy lives with sudden, swift power.

Lymphoma in dogs and cats is a manageable and treatable cancer. This book was written in an effort to provide a comprehensive guide to its diagnosis and treatment. It is my hope that you will find this book useful and that some good may come from its pages.

Contents

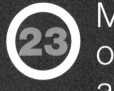

23 Management of self-harm and poisoning

I. Chukwulobelu and G. S. Seyan

Manor Hospital, Walsall, UK

Definition:
- Deliberate self-harm is an acute, non-fatal act carried out to cause harm
- Poisoning is taking a substance that causes health hazards. This can be done accidentally or deliberately, with the intention of self-harm or suicide

Incidence

- Deliberate self-harm has an annual incidence of 2–3/1000 people (rates are likely to be underestimated)
- Deliberate self-harm accounts for ~10% of all acute medical admissions in the UK
- Deliberate self-harm is more common in young females, with a worrying increase in incidence of 68% amongst girls aged 13–16 years since 2011
- Conversely, successful suicide attempts are more common in young males
- Self-poisoning accounts for 90% of medical presentations of deliberate self-harm
- Overdoses account for ~15% of acute medical emergencies
- Risk factors are listed in Box 23.1

Medical Student Survival Skills: The Acutely Ill Patient, First Edition. Philip Jevon, Konnur Ramkumar, and Emma Jenkinson.
© 2020 John Wiley & Sons Ltd. Published 2020 by John Wiley & Sons Ltd.
Companion website: www.wiley.com/go/jevon/medicalstudent

Box 23.1 Risk factors

Deliberate self-harm	Risk factors for suicide
Female	Male
History of mental health disease (personality disorders, autism)	History of mental health disease (especially depression and schizophrenia)
Triggering life events (e.g. abuse, unemployment, prison)	Prior suicide attempts (strongest predictive factor)
Lesbian, gay, bisexual, transgender, questioning (LGBTQ) population	Elderly population
Younger population	Chronic medical conditions (terminal and painful diseases)

Common risk factors

Low socioeconomic status
Alcohol abuse
Social isolation

Assessment and diagnosis of patients presenting with self-harm

History

- Ascertaining an accurate history may be difficult for the following reasons:
  - Reduced Glasgow coma score (GCS) as a result of poison
  - Altered mental state and psychosis as a result of poison
  - Inaccurate information as a result of an underlying mental health disorder
- Collateral history often provides invaluable information for discerning what drugs may have been taken and the circumstances around the overdose
- It is important to identify those with *genuine suicidal ideation* and those with risk of future self-harm. Features that indicate a genuine attempt are as follows:
  - Premeditation (preparation of a will, suicide notes, financial preparation)
  - Expected fatal outcome
  - Associated drug and alcohol use
  - Violent methods used
  - Precautions to discovery
  - Regret at failed attempt
- Suicide risk assessment tools are widely used in NHS trusts but have little evidence of being able to appropriately stratify patient risk; approximately 1% of patients presenting with self-harm will go on to commit suicide

- Overall clinical impression and intuition should not be ignored in the assessment of patients presenting with self-harm (Table 23.1)

NB Be aware!
Asking about suicidal ideation does not increase risk of suicide.

- Emergency treatment of poisoning should be according to Toxbase www.toxbase.org (username and password are available at each trust – if you do not know, ask in the emergency department)
- Toxbase is an invaluable resource that will provide detailed information on the toxins present in any formulae
- If any further information is required, contact your local poisons service or call the UK National Poisons Information Service on 0844 8920111

ABCDE approach to examination and management

Table 23.1 ABCDE approach to the examination and initial management of self-harm and poisoning

	Examine	Measure/monitor	Treat/intervention	Investigations
Airway	Assess for sounds of airway obstruction or compromise	O_2 saturations Capnography	Simple airway adjuncts if reduced GCS Contact anaesthetist if airway compromise (GCS <8)	
Breathing	Inspect, palpate, percuss, and auscultate Assess for any signs of aspiration	O_2 saturations – may appear cyanosed or flushed Respiratory rate – may have respiratory depression or tachypnoea If respiratory depression, consider naloxone 400 µg	High-flow oxygen (15 l min⁻¹) via non-rebreathe mask	Arterial blood gas (ABG) to assess for respiratory failure and metabolic acidosis (e.g. paracetamol, aspirin, and tricyclic antidepressant poisoning)

(Continued)

Table 23.1 (Continued)

	Examine	Measure/monitor	Treat/intervention	Investigations
Circulation	Inspect, palpate, and auscultate Check capillary refill and jugular venous pressure	Heart rate – may have tachycardia or bradycardia Blood pressure – may be hypotensive Urine output	Secure IV access – two wide bore cannulas Consider bolus fluids if hypotensive – e.g. 500 ml crystalloid stat Catheterise and monitor urine output – aim at 0.5 ml kg^{-1} h^{-1}	Bloods – full blood count, urea and electrolytes (U&Es), liver function tests (LFTs), clotting, ABG/venous blood gas Drug levels (paracetamol and salicylate) Electrocardiogram (ECG) – to look for specific pathology (e.g. broadening QRS in tricyclic depression overdose, ST elevation in cocaine use) Consider blood cultures Consider chest X-ray if signs of aspiration
Disability	Assess pupil size and response If reduced GCS then perform a full cranial nerve examination, and upper and lower limb neurological examination	Assess GCS Blood glucose (important for differentials)	Appropriate analgesia Blood glucose if <4 or >11 treat appropriately	Consider neuroimaging
Exposure	Assess for signs of IV drug use Check temperature Digital rectal examination or per vaginal examination to assess if patient has concealed drugs		Consider detaining patient under Mental Health Act if appropriate	Obtain collateral history Check Toxbase for specific management of poisoning

Poisoning

Principles of poisons management are as follows:

- Resuscitation of the patient
- Reducing the absorption of the poison if possible
- Giving specific antidotes if available (Table 23.2)

Table 23.2 Drug antidotes

Drug	Antidote
Beta-blockers	Glucagon, atropine
Benzodiazepines	Flumazenil if severe (use with caution)
Digoxin	Digibind
Ethylene glycerol	Fomepizole (better than ethanol)
Iron tablet	Desferrioxamine
Opiates	Naloxone

Common poisons include:
- Paracetamol
- Opiates
- Benzodiazepines
- Alcohol
- Antidepressants
- Aspirin

NB Be aware!
- 50% of patients will have also consumed alcohol
- 30% of patients will have taken multiple drugs

Signs and symptoms

Sign	Potential drug
Hypoventilation	Opiates, ethanol, benzodiazepines
Hyperventilation	Salicylic acid, carbon monoxide
Miosis	Opiates, acetylcholinergics
Dilated pupils	Anticholinergics
Bradycardia	Beta-blockers, digoxin
Tachyarrhythmias	Tricyclic antidepressants, lithium, cocaine
Hyperthermia	Ecstasy, amphetamines, SSRIs

Specific poisons

Paracetamol

In overdose, treatment is focused on restoring stores of glutathione to remove the toxic metabolite of paracetamol, *N*-acetyl-*p*-benzoquinone (NABQI).

- <24 hours: overdose symptoms are often mild and potentially asymptomatic
- 24–36 hours: right upper quadrant pain may have developed due to hepatic necrosis with associated signs of acute liver failure (jaundice, encephalopathy)
- Encephalopathy can worsen over the next 72 hours

Specific management

If the time of overdose is known then ideally blood levels should be taken at four hours post ingestion: once the levels are known then the following nomogram (Figure 23.1) is used to determine whether or not treatment should be commenced. Acetylcysteine should be commenced within eight hours of ingestion, therefore if there is any anticipated delay in obtaining blood levels before this time then treatment should be commenced whilst levels are pending.

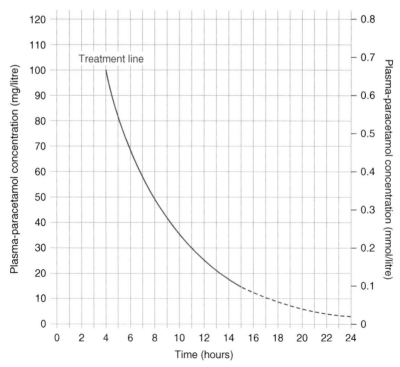

Figure 23.1 Treatment nomogram for paracetamol overdose (British National Formulary/Toxbase).

The following treatment regime should be used:

- First infusion: acetylcysteine 150 mg kg^{-1} in 200 ml 5% dextrose over 1 hour
- Second infusion: acetylcysteine 50 mg kg^{-1} in 500 ml 5% dextrose over 4 hours
- Third infusion: acetylcysteine 100 mg kg^{-1} in 1000 ml % dextrose over 16 hours. The 16 hourly infusion should continue until LFTs have been rechecked (seek senior advice)

NB Be aware!
In staggered paracetamol overdose (i.e. where tablets have been taken over a period of greater than one hour), blood levels are not useful for guiding the need for treatment, therefore acetylcysteine should be started immediately.

Liver transplantation
Indications for liver transplantation are according the King's College criteria (see Table 22.4):

- Arterial pH < 7.3, 24 hours after ingestion
- Or all of the following:
  - Prothrombin time (PT) > 100 seconds
  - Creatinine > 300 μmol l^{-1}
  - Grade III or IV encephalopathy

NB Be aware!
Remember patient trends and blood test trends are also important. Refer early if worsening PT, creatinine, or encephalopathy to allow the liver unit to assess and plan for a new patient.

Opiates

Overdosing usually occurs as a result of recreational use, but be wary of overdosing in patients who are opiate naïve or had dosing increased as part of chronic pain management.

Signs may include

- Respiratory depression is the cardinal feature of opioid toxicity (respiratory rate < 12)

- Pinpoint pupils (absence does not exclude possibility of toxicity)
- Reduced GCS
- Constipation

Specific management
- Initiate respiratory support using a bag–valve–mask if there are signs of severe respiratory depression (respiratory rate <8) and/or type respiratory failure on ABG
- Administer 400 μg of naloxone IV
  - IM and intranasal administration can be considered where IV access is not available, but they have unpredictable distribution profiles
  - The half-life of naloxone is shorter than opiates, so regular review is required
  - Giving enough naloxone to completely reverse the effects of opiates is *not* recommended. This can precipitate withdrawal symptoms and reverse pain control

NB Be aware!
Methadone and loperamide can cause prolonged QTc.

Aspirin (salicylic acid)

This is one of the most common drugs used in deliberate overdose. Moderate overdose patients present with the following:
- Tinnitus
- Epigastric pain
- Sweating
- Vomiting
- Blurring of vision

In adults a respiratory alkalosis initially develops as salicylic acid stimulates the central respiratory centres. A metabolic acidosis with a raised anion gap develops afterwards.

NB Be aware!
- Children are at risk of Reye's syndrome from taking aspirin – a condition that leads to encephalopathy and liver damage
- Children tend to only present with metabolic acidosis in aspirin overdose

Specific management
- Gastric lavage can be attempted within an hour of ingestion following large overdoses
- Urinary alkalinisation with sodium bicarbonate helps with elimination of aspirin, e.g. 1 L 1.26% $NaHCO_3$ with close monitoring of potassium
- Haemodialysis is indicated where there are the following:
  - Serum salicylate concentration > 700 mg l^{-1}
  - Metabolic acidosis refractory to treatment
  - Acute renal failure
  - Pulmonary oedema
  - Seizures
  - Coma

Tricyclic antidepressants

- Tricyclic antidepressants (TCAs) are highly toxic in overdose and can be fatal in doses 10× the daily dose
- Medications are lipophilic and protein bound so *cannot be dialysed*
- First generation TCAs are more likely to cause lethal intoxication
- Early signs are often related to the anticholinergic effects of TCAs:
  - Dry mouth
  - Dilated pupils
  - Tachycardia
  - Urinary retention

Specific management
- Patients with a reduced GCS should be managed in an intensive treatment unit (ITU) or high dependency unit (HDU) setting
- Gastric lavage and activated charcoal (50 g orally) should be given if the patient is seen with 1 hour of ingestion
- Ensure that an ECG is done on patients with suspected TCA poisoning
- Boluses of 50 mmol of 8.4% sodium bicarbonate IV should be given if there are either of the following:
  - Prolonged QRS duration
  - Metabolic acidosis

Selective serotonin reuptake inhibitors

- Common examples include fluoxetine, citalopram, and sertraline
- They are typically well tolerated in overdoses

- Ingestion of 30× the normal dose typically presents with minor or no symptoms at all. Ingestion of 50–75× the normal dose may cause vomiting and mild central nervous system depression
- Problems mainly arise when two serotonergics are ingested together, which may lead to 'serotonin syndrome'

Signs of serotonin syndrome
- Altered mental state
- Pyrexia
- Hyperreflexia
- Rigidity
- Dilated pupils
- Increased creatine kinase

Management of serotonin syndrome
- IV fluids
- Benzodiazepines
- In severe cases, give cyproheptadine

Cocaine

Cocaine is typically snorted or smoked (freebasing). This drug can present as massive overdosing when concealed packets (i.e. swallowed or per rectum) rupture; 1 g of pure cocaine is lethal.

Signs and symptoms
- Hypertension
- Pyrexia
- Agitation
- Seizures
- Tachycardia
- Chest pain

Complications
- Rhabdomyolysis
- Renal failure
- Psychosis
- Cerebrovascular events
- Myocardial infarction (related to vasospasm)

Specific management
- Give benzodiazepines to settle agitation
- Perform an ECG to look for any ischaemia and treat as an acute coronary syndrome or arrhythmias and treat according Resuscitation Council (UK) guidelines

Synthetic cannabinoids

These are a group of heterogeneous compounds that are designed to stimulate cannabinoid receptors. These compounds can range from two to 800 times more potent that their natural occurring counterparts. Initially designed to bypass drug legislation (now illegal), these drugs have seen a worrying increase of use in the twenty-first century.

Commonly known in the UK as Black Mamba its use is particularly prevalent amongst the homeless and prison populations. Given the variable nature of the compounds present, these drugs have the potential to cause serious and life-threatening toxicity.

Presentations of severe toxicity
- Florid toxic psychosis – similar to schizophrenia
- Coma
- Seizure
- Rhadomylosis
- Hyperthermia
- Respiratory arrest

Management
- Management is largely supportive
- ITU admission is common

Cardiopulmonary arrest

- Perform standard advanced life support (ALS)
- Give antidote/reversal agent if appropriate
- Consider magnesium sulphate if polymorphic VT (torsades de pointes) is the cause of the arrest

Prior to discharge

- Crisis team/psychiatric team input (check local policy)

OSCE Key Learning Points

✔ Consider poisoning in any unconscious adult with unknown cause

✔ Call for senior help early (SBAR)

✔ Refer to Toxbase for the specific management of poisons

✔ Staggered paracetamol overdose, start treatment without waiting for levels

24 Management of trauma

Background

- Trauma is the commonest cause of loss of life in those aged under 44 years
- Estimated to be second commonest cause of 'life years lost' to death/disability worldwide by 2020
- 10 000 people in England/Wales die from trauma each year
- The commonest cause of trauma in the UK is from road traffic collisions

Pathophysiology

- Depends on mechanism of injury (Box 24.1)
- It may involve systemic injury and/or specific organ injury
- *Immediate death* may occur due to asphyxia or exsanguination
- *Early deaths* occur due to failure to manage ABCDE problems
- *Late deaths* occur due to complications

Box 24.1 Types of trauma

- *Blunt trauma*: e.g. pedestrian hit by car, hit by baseball bat
- *Penetrating trauma*: e.g. gunshot wound, stabbing
- *Environmental trauma*: e.g. electrocution, burns, frostbite

Pre-hospital management and handover

- Most patients with significant trauma arrive by ambulance
- Ambulance staff should hand over using ATMIST (Box 24.2)
- Initial assessment/resuscitation will usually have begun pre-hospital

Medical Student Survival Skills: The Acutely Ill Patient, First Edition. Philip Jevon, Konnur Ramkumar, and Emma Jenkinson.
© 2020 John Wiley & Sons Ltd. Published 2020 by John Wiley & Sons Ltd.
Companion website: www.wiley.com/go/jevon/medicalstudent

Box 24.2 ATMIST handover

A	Age/sex of patient
T	Time of incident
M	Mechanism of injury
I	Injuries (found *or* suspected)
S	Signs – vital signs *and* trends (improving *or* deteriorating)
T	Treatment – what treatment has already been initiated?

Assessment

- The *primary survey* involves the assessment/treatment of immediately life-threatening problems using ABCDE
- The *secondary survey* is only commenced once the patient is stable – it involves a full head to toe assessment of the patient, aiming to detecting *all* injuries, however minor

Primary survey

- ABCDE approach (Box 24.3)
- Treat problems as you find them
- Reassessment is key

Box 24.3 Primary survey

A	Airway (with cervical spine control)
B	Breathing
C	Circulation
D	Disability
E	Environment/Exposure

Airway (with cervical spine control)

Assess the airway for:

- Visible obstructions (e.g. swelling, blood, foreign bodies)
- Noise (e.g. gurgling, stridor)
- *Potential* obstructions (e.g. singed hairs, carbon deposits, reduced conscious level)

Interventions

- Manual manoeuvres (e.g. chin lift, jaw thrust, *not* head tilt)
- Adjuncts (e.g. naso- or oropharyngeal airways)

NB

- The use of a nasopharyngeal airway is contraindicated in a potential base of skull fracture (i.e. patients with obvious head/facial injury)
- An oropharyngeal airway is unlikely to be tolerated in any patient not deeply unconscious (i.e. AVPU ≤ P (see Box 24.11), Glasgow coma score ≤ 8)

- Administer oxygen 15 l min⁻¹ via a non-rebreathe oxygen mask
- Definitive airway, e.g. ETT or surgical airway, is likely to require a specialist: call for help early

Manage the *cervical spine* with:

- Manual in-line immobilisation
- Consider triple immobilisation (with correctly fitting collar, blocks and tape) in patients where there is any doubt about the patient's ability to protect their own cervical spine, however exercise caution in patients with significant head injuries, where a tightly-fitting collar can worsen intracranial hypertension.

Breathing

Assess breathing (look, listen, feel) for:

- External signs of injury (wounds, bruising, deformity, tracheal deviation)
- Excursion (accessory muscle use, paradoxical movements)
- Decreased/absent air entry
- Tenderness/crepitus

Breathing problems that must be addressed

- Tension pneumothorax (Box 24.4) (needle thoracocentesis – Box 24.5)
- Open pneumothorax (three-way occlusive dressing – Box 24.6)

Box 24.4 Signs of tension pneumothorax

- Severe respiratory distress
- Pain
- Absence of breath sounds on affected side
- Hyperresonance on affected side
- Tachycardia
- Hypotension
- Tracheal deviation away from side of injury

Box 24.5 Needle thoracocentesis

- Landmark: 2nd intercostal space, mid-clavicular line (on affected side)
- Equipment: antiseptic swab, large bore needle
- Aiming to release the tension, i.e. convert to simple pneumothorax
- Must follow up with a chest drain as soon as possible

Box 24.6 Treatment of open pneumothorax

- Apply a non-adherent dressing and occlude it on *three* sides, not four

- Massive haemothorax (IV access and early chest drain – Box 24.7)
- Flail chest/pulmonary contusion (analgesia/early intubation)
- Cardiac tamponade (pericardiocentesis/early surgery)

Box 24.7 Treatment of massive haemothorax

- Get good intravenous access first
- Use open technique for chest drain insertion
- Use 'triangle of safety' (4–5th intercostal space, latissimus dorsi posteriorly, pectoralis major anteriorly, aiming anterior to mid-axillary line
- Ensure full personal protective equipment/sterile techniques
- Provide adequate analgesia/anaesthesia
- Make large skin incision insertion (immediately above rib, avoiding neurovascular bundle)
- Blunt dissect using artery forceps until through the pleura
- Finger-sweep to ensure there is no palpable liver, etc.
- Insert large drain using instrument, ensuring all holes are inside the chest
- Suture the drain securely
- Apply dressing to prevent accidental dislodging but allowing full view of incision site
- If patient drains > 1 l of blood discuss with thoracic surgeons as soon as possible

Circulation

Assess circulation (look, listen, feel) for:

- Heart sounds
- Pulse (volume/rate)
- Blood pressure
- Capillary refill time
- Signs of bleeding (chest, abdomen, pelvis, long bones, external bleeding)

Interventions

- Direct compression on bleeding wounds
- Compression on proximal arteries if above is not successful
- Application of tourniquet if above fails
- Adequate circulatory access (Box 24.8)
- Consideration of fluid requirement (e.g. 2 l crystalloid early if patient is shocked)
- Early consideration of blood (Box 24.9 – consider massive transfusion)

Box 24.8 Options for immediate access in trauma patients

- Intravenous (anterior cubital fossa or external jugular, hand or foot)
- Intraosseous (proximal tibial, distal femoral, proximal humerus)
- Central (subclavian, femoral, internal jugular)
- Venous cut-down (long saphenous vein)

Box 24.9 Options for blood requesting

- O-negative (immediately available if required)
- Type specific (ABO matched – takes ~15 minutes)
- Fully cross matched (takes ~1 hour)
- Massive transfusion pack (packed red blood cells plus clotting factors)

Disability

Assess disability for:

- Alterations in conscious level (AVPU – Box 24.10)
- Pupillary response to light and accommodation
- Obvious lateralising signs or focal neurology

Box 24.10 AVPU scale

- **A**lert
- Responds to **V**oice
- Responds to **P**ain
- **U**nresponsive

Exposure/Environment

- External signs of injury
- Environmental factors (remove chemicals/heat, rewarm, etc.)
- Check blood sugar and core temperature, if not already done

Special populations

- Elderly (different physiology/pharmacology)
- Paediatric (different psychology/physiology, distressed parents)
- Obstetric (different physiology, slightly altered priorities)
- Athletes (different physiology)

Secondary survey

- Thjs only takes place once the primary survey is completed and the patient is stabilised
- Take an 'AMPLE' history (Box 24.11) and head to toe examination
- Timing and adjuncts will depend on the patient and facilities

Box 24.11 AMPLE history

A	Allergies
M	Medications
P	Past medical history/pregnancy
L	Last meal
E	Events surrounding incident

Avoiding complications

The following simple things can be done to avoid late complications:
- Avoid hypoxia
- Maintain normovolaemia
- Normalise $PaCO_2$
- Minimise risk of raised intracranial pressure
- Avoid hypothermia
- Consider early administration of clotting factors

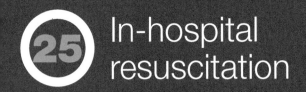

In-hospital resuscitation

25

NB Try to prevent cardiac arrest – 80% of patients who have a cardiac arrest in hospital display adverse signs prior to collapse.

- Cardiopulmonary resuscitation (CPR) is an emergency procedure performed during a cardiac arrest in an attempt to re-establish circulation and breathing
- The Resuscitation Council (UK) in-hospital algorithm (Figure 25.1) provides guidance for in-hospital resuscitation
- CPR is performed to keep a patient alive until a reversible cause can be treated and advanced emergency care can be provided
- With most patients displaying adverse signs prior to cardiac arrest, the recognition of acute illness, together with effective treatment and appropriate management following the ABCDE approach to prevent deterioration is paramount

Procedure

Safety

- Ensure it is safe to approach
- Don gloves, aprons, etc. as soon as it is practical to do so
- Check for and remove hazards, e.g. bed table, trailing electrical cables, IV fluids stand
- Remember the Resuscitation Council (UK) guidelines for safer handling in resuscitation

Medical Student Survival Skills: The Acutely Ill Patient, First Edition. Philip Jevon, Konnur Ramkumar, and Emma Jenkinson.
© 2020 John Wiley & Sons Ltd. Published 2020 by John Wiley & Sons Ltd.
Companion website: www.wiley.com/go/jevon/medicalstudent

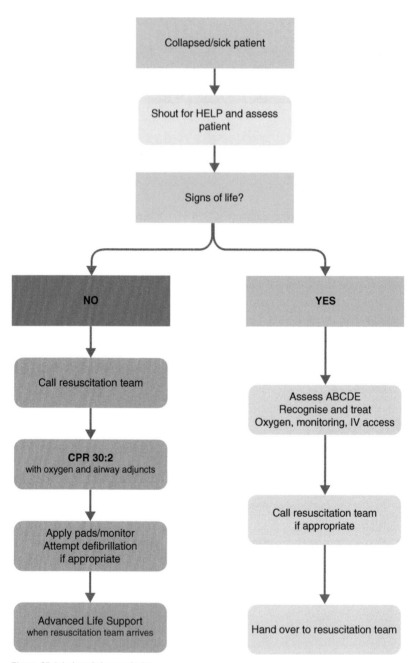

Figure 25.1 In-hospital resuscitation.

Check for response

- Gently shake the shoulders and ask loudly, 'Are you all right?' (Figure 25.2)
- If the patient responds, reassess following the ABCDE approach (see Chapter 1)
- If the patient does not respond, call out for help/pull the emergency buzzer (Figure 25.3), get the patient flat, open the airway, and check for signs of normal breathing

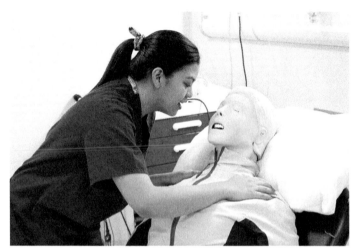

Figure 25.2 Check for responsiveness.

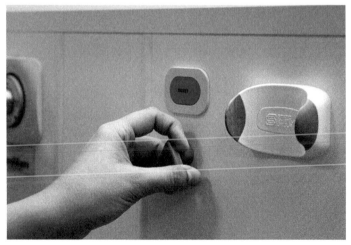

Figure 25.3 Summon help from colleagues.

Check for signs of life

- Open the airway: head tilt/chin lift (jaw thrust if cervical spine injury is suspected)
- Look, listen, and feel for signs of normal breathing for no longer than 10 seconds (Figure 25.4)

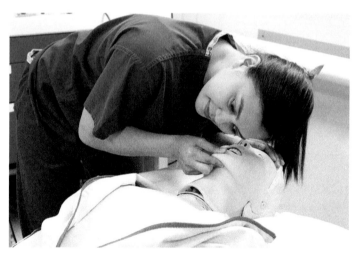

Figure 25.4 Perform head tilt/chin lift and check for signs of normal breathing.

 Common mistakes and pitfalls

Agonal breathing (occasional gasps, slow, laboured, or noisy breathing) is common in the first few minutes following a cardiac arrest. Do not mistake this for normal breathing.

- If the patient is breathing normally, perform ABCDE assessment, call for help, and escalate if necessary. Consider using the recovery position
- If the patient is not breathing normally, start chest compressions while colleagues alert the cardiac arrest team and fetch a cardiac arrest trolley and defibrillator

Alert the cardiac arrest team

- Alert the cardiac arrest team following local protocols. This usually involves calling 2222 and advising the switchboard of the emergency (cardiac arrest) and location (Figure 25.5)

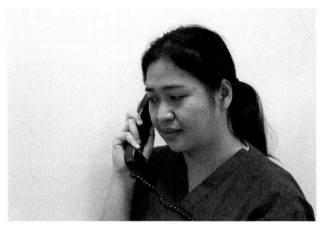

Figure 25.5 Summon cardiac arrest team: usually call 2222.

- Ensure the cardiac arrest team have access – sometimes access doors may be security locked

Chest compressions
- Ensure the bed is at a suitable height to perform chest compressions. The patient should be level with the rescuer's knee to mid-thigh region
- Place the heel of one hand on the centre of the patient's chest and the heel of the other hand on top; interlock the fingers, lifting them off the rib cage
- Ensure your arms are straight, elbows locked, and start performing chest compressions at a rate of 100–120 min⁻¹ at a depth of 5–6 cm (Figure 25.6)

NB Allow the chest to completely recoil after each compression otherwise venous return can be compromised.

- Ensure chest compression/relaxation times are approximately equal and minimise interruptions to chest compressions
- Deliver chest compressions to ventilations at a ratio of 30 : 2 (Figure 25.7). In-hospital chest compressions are typically performed continuously until a self-inflating bag device is available for ventilations

Ventilations
- As soon as the self-inflating bag arrives, attach oxygen at a flow rate of 10–15 l min⁻¹ and ideally insert an airway device, e.g. oropharyngeal airway or i-gel (more experienced practitioners may insert a tracheal tube)

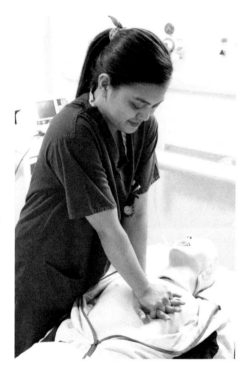

Figure 25.6 Perform chest compressions.

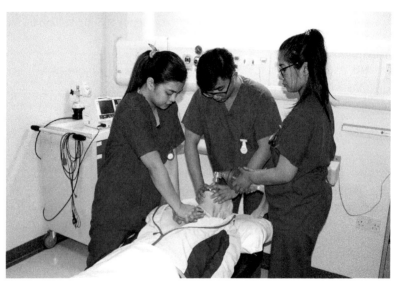

Figure 25.7 CPR: 30 chest compressions to 2 ventilations.

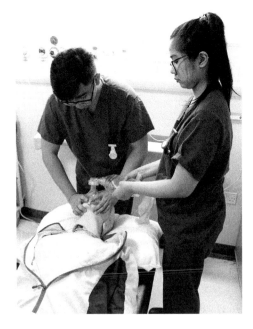

Figure 25.8 Two person technique for bag–valve–mask ventilation.

- Ensure the airway is open and there is an adequate seal between the mask and the patient's mouth (Figure 25.8)
- Stop chest compressions and deliver two ventilations, each over 1 second and then continue chest compressions and ventilations at a ratio of 30:2

Defibrillation (if required)

- Once the defibrillator arrives, switch it on, and use in automated external defibrillator (AED) mode
- Attach large adhesive defibrillation pads to the patient's bare chest – one to the right of the sternum below the clavicle and the other in the mid-axillary line approximately level with the V6 electrocardiogram (ECG) electrode, avoiding breast tissue

NB Chest compressions should continue while pads are being attached.

- Once the defibrillator starts to analyse the ECG, ensure cadiopulmonary resuscitation (CPR) is stopped. If a shock is required the defibrillator will charge up and advise you to shock (semi-automatic)

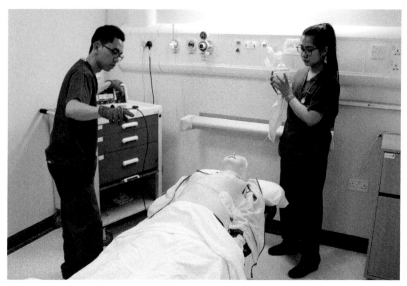

Figure 25.9 Automated external defibrillation: ensure everyone is clear of the patient.

- Before pressing the shock button, ensure everyone is clear of the patient and that the oxygen is removed 1 m (Figure 25.9)
- After delivering the shock continue with CPR for 2 minutes

Cardiac arrest rhythms – shockable

Ventricular fibrillation

- In ventricular fibrillation (VF) various groups of cells within the ventricles are depolarising and repolarising in an uncoordinated, random, and chaotic way
- This results in insufficient contraction of the left ventricle and insufficient cardiac output to produce a pulse

Ventricular tachycardia

- In ventricular tachycardia (VT) cells within the ventricles are initiating the action potential at a fast rate, usually 120–200 bpm
- In some cases this rate may be so fast that it does not allow sufficient time for adequate ventricular filling, resulting in a reduction in cardiac output. If this reduction is dramatic enough, the casualty may not have a palpable pulse; the rhythm is described as 'pulseless ventricular tachycardia'

Cardiac arrest rhythms – non-shockable

Asystole

- Asystole is often described as a 'straight line'. However, in reality the line is rarely (if ever) straight
- Occasionally P waves may be seen
- This rhythm is known by a number of different names including ventricular standstill and P wave asystole

Pulseless electrical activity

- Pulseless electrical activity (PEA) occurs in patients who have organised cardiac electrical activity in the absence of any palpable pulses
- There will always be an underlying cause to PEA

Potentially reversible causes: The four 'H's and four 'T's

Potentially reversible or aggravating causes for the cardiac arrest should be considered and where possible appropriate treatment initiated. The main reversible causes are identified as the four 'H's and four 'T's, using their initial letter.

- Hypoxia
- Hypovolaemia
- Hyperkalaemia, hypokalaemia, hypoglycaemia, hypocalcaemia, acidaemia, and other metabolic disorders
- Hypothermia
- Tension pneumothorax
- Tamponade
- Toxins
- Thrombosis (pulmonary or coronary)

Hypoxia

- Any casualty in cardiac arrest will have some degree of hypoxia
- Oxygen should be administered using as high a concentration as possible
- Check regularly to make sure that any oxygen tubing used is connected securely to the oxygen flow meter

- Oxygen cylinders found on many cardiac arrest trolleys have limited capacity. Check the cylinder pressure gauge regularly to ensure that the cylinder is not empty
- Always use a central supply of oxygen via an outlet in the wall by the casualty's bed whenever possible

Hypovolaemia

- Hypovolaemia is usually due to severe haemorrhage. Intravenous fluids should be administered rapidly and, if necessary, arrangements made for urgent surgery
- Although there has been a great deal of debate as to the most appropriate fluids to give in such circumstances, it is suggested that there is no advantage in using a colloid so either sodium chloride 0.9% or Hartmann's solution should be used

Hyperkalaemia, hypokalaemia, and other metabolic disorders

- The casualty's medical history may suggest an abnormality, with appropriate tests confirming the levels
- Treatment should be directed at returning any abnormal values to normal limits; 10 ml of 10% calcium chloride or calcium gluconate can be used in the presence of hyperkalaemia and hypocalcaemia

Hypothermia

- If hypothermia is suspected, the casualty's body temperature must be checked using a low reading thermometer. Hypothermia is defined as a core body temperature below 35 °C and is further classified as being mild (32–35 °C), moderate (30–32 °C), or severe (< 30 °C)
- Emphasis is placed on rewarming the casualty, whilst maintaining CPR throughout. Various options are available for use for a patient in cardiac arrest including warming intravenous fluids, and placing warm fluid into the casualty's bladder, peritoneal (abdominal) cavity, or pleural (thoracic) cavity
- Many drugs and other treatment options such as defibrillation may be ineffective at temperatures below 30 °C and careful consideration needs to be given to the use of these at such low temperatures

Tension pneumothorax

- A tension pneumothorax may be the result of trauma to the chest, a severe asthma attack, positive pressure ventilation, including the use of a bag-valve-mask, or following some medical procedures such as the insertion of a central venous line

- Initial management of a tension pneumothorax involves the insertion of a large bore cannula into the 2nd intercostal space in the mid-clavicular line (needle thoracocentesis). The casualty will also require the insertion of a chest drain

Tamponade

- A cardiac tamponade results from fluid or blood entering the pericardial space. As more fluid enters the space, more pressure is exerted on the heart until it is physically unable to beat, resulting in little or no cardiac output
- A cardiac tamponade is difficult to diagnose, especially during a cardiac arrest. A cardiac tamponade should be considered in any casualty in cardiac arrest following penetrating chest trauma, and chest or cardiac surgery. A needle pericardiocentesis should be considered

Toxins

- Consideration should be given to the possibility that the casualty has a specific history of accidental or deliberate poisoning. Specific antidotes may be available
- Many hospital emergency departments have databases outlining the appropriate treatment options for many drugs, plants, or other chemicals and toxic substances that may be ingested. Similarly, the National Poisons Information Service (www.npis.org) offers such advice
- CPR must be continued in the pulseless casualty whilst any other treatment is undertaken

Thrombosis

- The most likely cause is a large pulmonary embolism
- Thrombolytic drugs should be considered. However, thrombolytic drugs may take up to 90 minutes to be effective and must only be used if it is appropriate to continue resuscitative attempts for this duration

References

Bernal, W., Auzinger, G., Dhawan, A., and Wendon, J. (2010). Acute liver failure. *Lancet* 376: 190–201.

Blatchford, O., Murray, W.R., and Blatchford, M. (2000). A risk score to predict need for treatment for upper gastrointestinal haemorrhage. *Lancet* 356 (9238): 1318–1321.

Rockall, T.A., Logan, R.F., Devlin, H.B., and Northfield, T.C. (1996). Risk assessment after acute upper gastrointestinal haemorrhage. *Gut* 38 (3): 316–321.

Rutherford, R.B. (2009). Clinical staging of acute limb ischaemia as the basis for choice of revascularization method: when and how to intervene. *Seminars in Vascular Surgery* 22 (1): 5–9.

Slack, A. and Wendon, J. (2011). Acute liver failure. *Clinical Medicine* 11 (3): 254–258.

Index

Note: Page numbers in *italics* refer to figures.
Page numbers in **bold** refer to tables.

Medical Student Survival Skills: The Acutely Ill Patient, First Edition. Philip Jevon,
Konnur Ramkumar, and Emma Jenkinson.
© 2020 John Wiley & Sons Ltd. Published 2020 by John Wiley & Sons Ltd.
Companion website: www.wiley.com/go/jevon/medicalstudent

I)

Non-Cutaneous Lymphoma

Lymphoma is a common and usually treatable malignancy of dogs and cats. Although there are many similarities in the disease manifestations in these species, there are significant and important differences in their cause, clinical presentations, and their response to treatment. My purpose is to explore the similarities and differences of lymphoma in dogs and cats and to present the clinician with a comprehensive overview of current standards of diagnosis and treatment.

Incidence and Prevalance

When evaluating the literature about lymphoma, you will encounter the terms *incidence* and *prevalence*. These terms are not the same and there is confusion about them. They are sometimes erroneously used interchangeably. Incidence refers the frequency of a disease in a population occurring over a defined period of time (usually one year) divided by the total population at risk.

Prevalence refers to the frequency of a disease in a population occurring at the same time divided by the number of individuals in the exposed population.

DOG

Lymphoma is one of the most common malignancies in dogs. Reported annual rates of occurrence range between 6 and 30 cases per 100,000 dogs per year.[1,2] In 2002, one estimate of the numbers of dogs in the United States was 60.7 million.[3] This suggests a range of 3,342 to 18,210 cases of lymphoma occurred in dogs that year. Breeds reported to experience a higher than average prevalence include boxers, Scottish terriers, basset hounds, Airedale terriers, chow chows, German shepherds, poodles, St. Bernards, English bulldogs, beagles, and golden retrievers. Rate of occurrence increases with age.[1]

CAT

Lymphoma is the most common malignancy reported in cats and it accounts for approximately one third of all tumors occurring in this species. In early surveys of cats with lymphoma, the estimated rate of occurrence was between 160 and 200 cases per 100,000 cats.[1,4] In 2002, the estimate of the population of cats in the United States was 76.8 million.[3] This suggests that between 122,880 and 153,600 cases of lymphoma should occur in cats each year. It is not clear if the rate of occurrence has remained the same as indicated in earlier studies or if it has changed following the introduction and wide spread use of vaccinations against feline leukemia virus (FeLV) infection. The current prevalence of lymphoma in the general population of cats is unknown. It seems very likely that lymphoma may now occur less often in the general cat population because of the wide spread use of FeLV vaccines. However, it may also be that too small a percentage of the entire cat population is vaccinated in any one year to change the overall prevalence of FeLV associated disorders including lymphoma.[5]

Etiology

DOG

The cause(s) of lymphoma in dogs is unknown. There have been several reports that at first seemed to incriminate a particular etiology but that were later proven to be false. Among these false reports of causes of canine lymphoma are exposure to phenoxay-acetic acid herbicide (2,4-D) on the lawns of their owners and exposure to low frequency magnetic fields created by electric currents and electric transmission lines.[6,7] Based on uncommon reports of lymphoma developing in related pure breed dogs, it is possible that genetics plays a more prominent role in tumor development in some dogs than in others. Dogs with lymphoma have a chromosomal segregation error that may promote or not interfere with malignant transformation.[8]

Interestingly, the canine MYC gene has the same structural organization as the human MYC gene, and the IGH, TCRB, and BCL2 genes of dogs also show organizational similarities to humans. Activation of MYC and BCL2 protooncogenes from chromosome translocation has been shown to be a major pathway in the development of non-Hodgkin's lymphoma in humans (protooncogenes are normal cellular genes that, when transformed or mutated, code for malignant phenotype and become known as oncogenes). A similar mechanism may occur in dogs that develop lymphoma.[9] In addition, c-N-ras mutations are uncommon in dogs and humans with lymphoma further suggesting the potential for a similar etiologic pathway to humans.[10] Unlike in cats, a viral etiology has not been established in dogs.

CAT

The only documented cause of lymphoma in cats is FeLV. Until the 1990's approximately 70% of cats with lymphoma in the United States and Western Europe were FeLV positive. In a very recent study from the Netherlands only 4 of 54 cats were FeLV positive. Similarly, reports from the 1980's suggested that 75%-85% of cats with mediastinal lymphoma would test positive for FeLV, but in this study from the Netherlands only 18.8% of cats with mediastinal lymphoma were FeLV test positive.[4] These findings raise new questions about the exclusive role of FeLV in causing lymphoma in cats especially in geographic areas with low FeLV prevalence like the Netherlands.

Another recent survey of FeLV status in Australian cats with lymphoma found that only 2 of 107 cats (2%) were serum FeLV test positive (ELISA). In contrast, 25 of 97 tumors (26%) tested were found to contain FeLV DNA after polymerase chair reaction (PCR) amplification of FeLV provirus (166 base pair segments of the FeLV U3 long terminal repeat). This suggests that factors other than FeLV are responsible for the development of lymphoma in at least some Australian cats. [10a]

There are several case reports that document cats developing lymphoma after treatment for a vaccine-associated sarcoma. Vaccine-associated sarcoma is not associated with the presence of FeLV. It is not clear what, if any, is the basis for this rare association of lymphoma with vaccine-associated sarcoma. [10b, 10c]

FeLV affects cats worldwide, but the prevalence of disease varies with geographic location. FeLV is transmitted cat to cat through intimate contact with saliva or body fluids (usually licking, grooming, biting, sharing food or water bowls and sharing litter pans). The virus can also be transmitted in milk to kittens and by blood transfusions.[11]

Fleas are an important vector in the transmission of a number of pathogens, such as bacteria and rickettsiae and perhaps FeLV as well. A new investigation of the role of the cat flea (*Centocephalides felis*) in the spread of FeLV raised several interesting issues regarding transmission of FeLV.[12] In this study, FeLV RNA could be detected in fleas and in their feces after being fed FeLV positive cat blood for 24 hours. This finding raises the possible risk of a healthy cat scratching flea feces into its skin as the result of pruritic flea bites or while fighting with other cats. It also raises the possibility of direct transmission of FeLV through the flea and flea bites.[12]

FeLV belongs to a family of viruses known as retroviruses (retroviridae) and to the subfamily oncornavirus (oncovirinae), or tumor-producing RNA viruses. Like other retroviruses, it contains a single strand of RNA and an enzyme called reverse transcriptase (RT). It is the RT enzyme that allows the virus to transform the cats normal DNA because it allows the viral RNA to be used as a template for new DNA production instead of the normal host DNA. FeLV is usually considered to be the cause of lymphoma in both FeLV test-positive and FeLV test-negative cats.[1,11,13,14]

After oral and or nasal exposure has occurred, the virus replicates in the tonsils and pharyngeal lymph nodes (2-4 days post exposure). At this stage, many cats mount an adequate immune response, reject the virus, and become immune. Cats that do not mount an adequate immune response become persistently infected and the virus infects a small number of circulating lymphocytes and monocytes (1-14 days post exposure). These infected cells then replicate in bone marrow neutrophils, platelet precursors, and intestinal crypt epithelium (7-21 days post exposure). FeLV replication in bone marrow proceeds rapidly and marrow origin neutrophils and platelets, or even free virus can establish a viremia (14-28 days post exposure). FeLV then spreads to various tissues and the cycle of infection is completed when infectious FeLV is shed in the saliva and, less important, urine or feces.[11]

Three different outcomes can result once a susceptible cat has been infected with FeLV. Some cats mount an immune response, neutralize the virus, and become resistant to future infections. These cats are sometimes referred to in the literature as "recovered" or "regressors" because the disease regresses. This happens in about 40% of exposed cats.[11]

Alternatively, after an initial period of viremia and virus shedding, a cat can test FeLV negative, but still harbor the virus in a latent form. These cats are sometimes called "latent carriers" and they are neither recovered nor acutely infected, but they are susceptible to developing clinical disease in the future. Depending on the cat's age at the time of infection and presumably on its immune status, up to 30% of exposed cats are in this category.[11]

The last possibility is that a cat becomes persistently viremic and sheds virus and progress to develop clinical disease associated with FeLV. About 30% of exposed cats will develop clinical disease and about 83% of these will die within 3 years. These cats are often referred to as "progressors" because of the progressive nature of their disease.[11]

FeLV Testing

Enzyme-linked immuno-sorbent assay (ELISA) is the most common testing method used for detecting transient and persistent FeLV infections. The principle of ELISA testing for FeLV relies on the detection of the p27 antigen (a core protein of the virus). ELISA testing can detect p27 in whole blood, serum, plasma, tears, or saliva. While ELISA testing on tears and or saliva can be done, such fluids are known to result in disproportionate false negative and false positive test results and are not recommended.[13]

Immunofluorescent antibody (IFA) testing detects the presence of structural antigen within the cytoplasm of infected leukocytes and platelets. Both FeLV testing systems assay for viral antigens and do not measure the immune response. The ELISA test is generally preferred as a screening test and the IFA test is generally reserved for use as a confirmatory test for FeLV. A validated IFA test should always be run to confirm results on a healthy ELISA positive cat before considering it viremic. A positive IFA is diagnostic of persistent bone marrow-origin viremia. Performed properly, 98% of IFA positive cats are also positive on viral isolation. Rare discordant results between IFA and virus isolation are likely due to early infection, prior to full bone marrow infection.[14]

Testing should occur before any new cat or kitten is introduced into a single or a multiple cat household to prevent exposure of the pre-existing household cats. Newly adopted cats and kittens should also be tested even if they represent the only cats in the household. If the FeLV status of a cat in an existing household is unknown, it should be tested because cats with FeLV can be asymptomatic for years while exposing other cats. FeLV testing should also be done on any cat that has potential recent exposure regardless of previous negative test results because FeLV status can change. Any sick cat should be evaluated for FeLV because the virus is associated with a wide variety of clinical illness. Cats presented for FeLV vaccination should be tested to establish their FeLV status prior to vaccination.[13]

Discordant results are defined as conflicting test results, usually between and ELISA positive and an IFA negative result. Discordancy can result due to testing in the early phase of infection; antigenemia without viremia (no intact virus); or a false positive ELISA due to faulty technique or cross-reactive antigens. These cats should be monitored by both ELISA and IFA assays at 4 to 8 week intervals for at lest 90 days.[13]

Annual testing of cats at risk is advised. Cats at risk are those with known or potential exposure to FeLV including: outdoor cats, fighting cats, strays, cats with bite wounds, escapees, recently mated females if the FeLV status of the male is unknown, cats in open multiple-cat households, cats in closed multiple-cat households with any cats of unknown FeLV status, cats in households having a known FeLV positive cat.[13]

Kittens can be tested at any age and maternal immunity in young kittens does not interfere with FeLV tests. In addition, vaccination against FeLV does not interfere with FeLV testing because the diagnostic tests assay for viral antigens and are not a measure of a cat's immune response to vaccination. See Figure 1 for a summary of recommendations for FeLV testing from the American Associations of Feline Practitioners and the Academy of Feline Medicine.[13]

Latent FeLV infections in which proviral DNA is present in a non-replicating form in bone marrow derived myelomonocytic progenitor cells have been suspected to be associated with diseases such as lymphoma, leukemia, and cytopenias. Latent FeLV infections are undetectable with ELISA or IFA testing. Many cats with what are regarded as "FeLV associated diseases," are test negative on traditional FeLV assays. PCR is advocated by some as an alternative to ELISA testing and as a means to detect FeLV proviral DNA in bone marrow of cats suspected of having latent infection. Recent studies of PCR for this purpose has raised questions related to historical assumptions.

PCR is a technology that allows for the detection and identification of very small bits of DNA or RNA within a given sample by creating relatively large amounts of identical material. The reaction mixture contains the sample to be analyzed, a bacterial derived polymerase, oligonucleotide primers that are complementary to the 3' and 5' ends of the DNA (or RNA) sequence to be analyzed and cofactors that assist the enzymatic reactions. A programmable heat block alternately heats the sample and denatures the nucleic acid (separates the double-strand nucleic acid to single-strand) in the sample during the heating phase, and cools the sample and anneals the oligonucleotide primers to the complementary regions of the unknown nucleic acid. Heat stable polymerases in the reaction mixture, using the strands to which the primers are annealed as a template, synthesize two double-stranded DNA copies for every molecule of double-stranded DNA in the original mixture. At the end of one cycle, the quantity of the original unknown sample has doubled. After x number of cycles, you can create 2^x molecules that are identical to the original single template.[15,16]

In a study that included 16 cats suspected to have latent FeLV infection, PCR, ELISA, and IFA on bone marrow were performed and

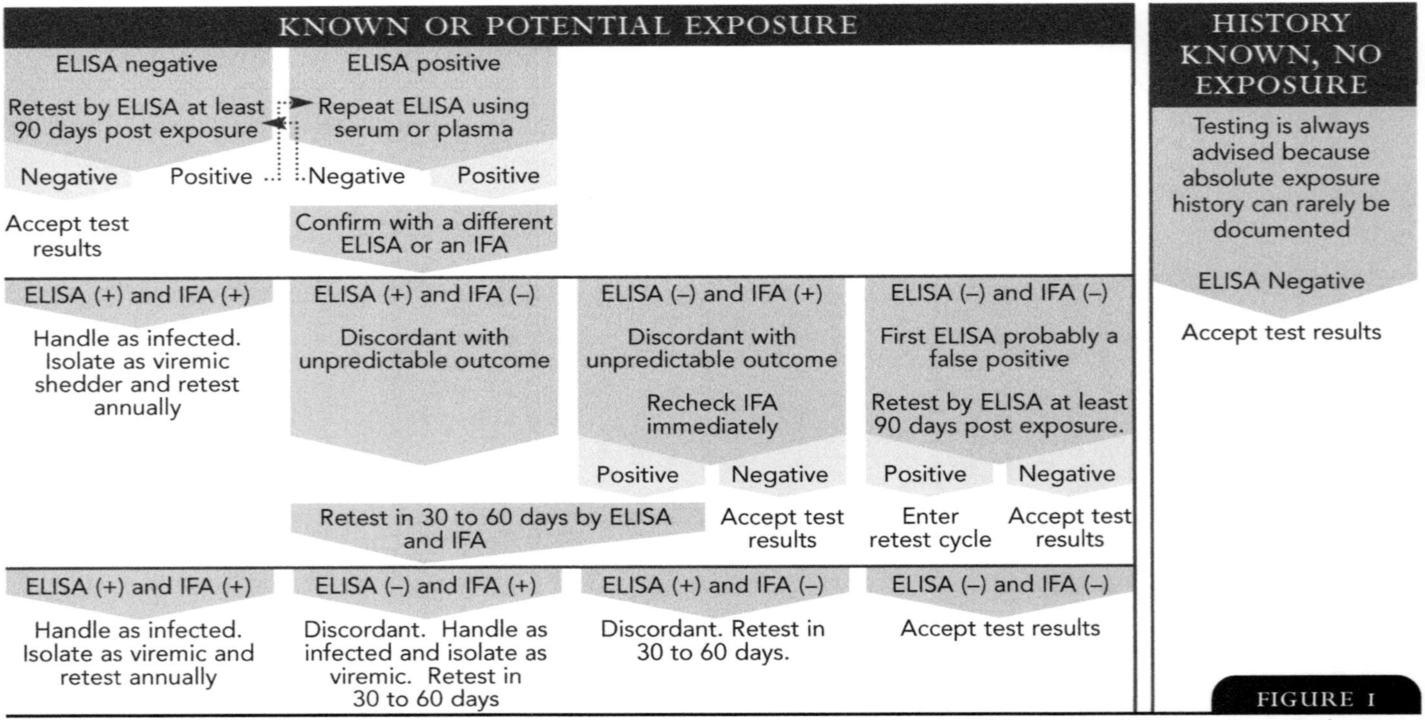

HISTORY KNOWN, NO EXPOSURE

Testing is always advised because absolute exposure history can rarely be documented

ELISA Negative → Accept test results

KNOWN OR POTENTIAL EXPOSURE

ELISA negative → Retest by ELISA at least 90 days post exposure
- Negative → Accept test results
- Positive → Repeat ELISA using serum or plasma
  - Negative
  - Positive → Confirm with a different ELISA or an IFA

ELISA positive

ELISA (+) and IFA (+): Handle as infected. Isolate as viremic shedder and retest annually

ELISA (+) and IFA (-): Discordant with unpredictable outcome. Retest in 30 to 60 days by ELISA and IFA
- ELISA (+) and IFA (+): Handle as infected. Isolate as viremic and retest annually
- ELISA (+) and IFA (-): Discordant. Handle as infected and isolate as viremic. Retest in 30 to 60 days
- ELISA (-) and IFA (+): Discordant. Retest in 30 to 60 days → Recheck IFA immediately
  - Positive → Enter retest cycle
  - Negative → Accept test results
- ELISA (-) and IFA (-): First ELISA probably a false positive. Retest by ELISA at least 90 days post exposure.
  - Positive → Enter retest cycle
  - Negative → Accept test results

ELISA (-) and IFA (-): Accept test results

FIGURE 1

Suggested FeLV Testing Plan for Healthy Cats. Whenever accepting negative FelV test results, be sure to test again following any subsequent exposure. Final testing should be done at least 90 days post-exposure. Cats may be retested earlier than the 90 days, but for the most confidence in the testing results, retests should be done at least 90 after exposure. (Modified from Edwards, D, Elston T, Loar, A, et al. Recommendations for feline retrovirus testing. American Association of Feline Practitioners and the Academy of Feline Medicine, 1997.)

compared.[14] These cats had disorders such as pancytopenia, leukopenia, neutropenia, non-regenerative anemia, lymphoma, and different types of leukemia that have historically been attributed to latent FeLV infection. In this study 12 of the 16 cats were negative on serum ELISA, blood and bone marrow IFA, and blood and bone marrow PCR. None of the 16 cats were test positive on bone marrow PCR alone. It appears that persistent or latent FeLV infection is not always present (detectable?) in conditions classically associated with FeLV.[14] This is an important observation because it forces the conclusion that FeLV may not always be the cause of what have been previously described as FeLV associated diseases.

Vaccination for FeLV

Vaccination does not affect the FeLV carrier state or the development of disease in cats with existing infection. Existing carriers remain a risk to other unexposed cats even after vaccination, and an existing carrier cat can subsequently become ill and appear to be a "vaccination failure."[13]

The routine vaccination of cats can result in inflammatory granuloma formation at the site of injection, and some of these will progress to sarcoma. Sarcomas that develop at vaccination sites are referred to as vaccine-associated sarcomas (VAS). Most reported VASs have followed rabies vaccination, but they are also reported secondary to vaccination for FeLV (and other immunizations and injections in cats). The prevalence of VAS is unknown, but best estimates put it somewhere between 1 case per 1,000 vaccinations and 1 case per 10,000 vaccinations.[17]

The American Association of Feline Practitioners (AAFP) and the Academy of Feline Medicine (AFM) considers FeLV vaccines to be either core or non-core to feline health programs. Core vaccinations are those recommended for every cat, while the need for non-core vaccinations will depend on the individual circumstances and risk factors present. Vaccination against FeLV is **recommended** for cats that are not restricted to a closed indoor environment that is free of the virus. Vaccination against FeLV infection is most important for cats living in these environmental criteria that are less than

16 weeks of age, but it is not recommended for cats 16 weeks or older with minimal to no risk of exposure. In addition, vaccinations for FeLV infections are not advised any more frequently than every three years.[13]

Histologic Classification

A number of histologic classification schemes based on microscopic appearance that have been used to grade lymphoma in humans have been adopted for use in veterinary pathology and oncology. Older classification schemes used in human and veterinary oncology include the Rappaport scheme and the Kiel scheme (an updated Kiel classification scheme remains the standard in Europe). Major differences between animal and human lymphomas exist such as animals having a higher proportion of high grade lymphomas than is observed in people and Hodgkin-like tumors are rarely identified in animals.[18]

Unfortunately, there still is no universal standard among veterinary pathologists by which a lymphoid tumor is classified. Clinicans in North America may receive histopathology reports from pathologists that diagnose lymphoma and classify it according to the Rappaport, Kiel, or NCI-WF systems. On the other hand, clinicians in North America are just as likely to receive reports that simply diagnose lymphoma and make no effort at providing additional classification data. The entire topic of the histologic classification of lymphoid malignancies in veterinary medicine remains unsettled and is in the process of transition.

The classification scheme developed by the National Cancer Institute called the Working Formulation (NCI-WF) can be applied to dogs and cats with lymphoma and is a more useful system than earlier schemes (Table 1). The NCI-WF uses mitotic index and natural rate of progression to classify tumors as low-, intermediate-, or high-grade. High-grade tumors are populated by large lymphoblasts with abundant cytoplasm and high mitotic activity. High-grade tumors are rapidly progressive clinically and can be either B- or T-cell type. Low-grade tumors are populated by small

TABLE 1
NCI WORKING FORMULATION CLASSIFICATION OF LYMPHOMA
Low-grade
Small lymphocytic, consistent with chronic lymphocytic leukemia
Follicular, predominantly small cleaved cell
Follicular, mixed small cleaved and large cell
Intermediate-grade
Follicular, predominantly large cell
Diffuse, small cleaved cell
Diffuse mixed, small and large cell
Diffuse, large cell cleaved or noncleaved cell
High-grade
Immunoblastic, large cell
Lymphoblastic, convoluted or non-convoluted cell
Small non-cleaved cell, Burkitt's or non-Burkitt's

cells with a low mitotic rate. Low-grade tumors are more slowly progressive clinically and are usually B-cell type.[18]

Prior to the adoption of the NCI-WF there were several different histologic classification systems in use that had been adopted from human medicine and this resulted in confusion among pathologists and oncologists.[1,19] As the authors of a recent comprehensive review of lymphoma in domestic animals have explained: *The major confusion caused by the veterinary use of human classifications is the definition of the terms "lymphoblast" and "lymphoblastic lymphoma." In human pathology, the term "lymphoblast" indicates an immature cell of small size that is able to divide but is larger than a mature lymphocyte and smaller than a large lymphocyte. In veterinary literature, it has been common to refer to the largest malignant lymphocytes as lymphoblasts. Consequently, the specific aggressive small-cell lymphoma termed "lymphoblastic" in human systems was largely unrecognized in animals. The importance of this distinction is that lymphoblastic lymphoma in the NCI-WF context is a clinical and diagnostic entity in dogs and cats, like the human counterpart, follows a short course and responds poorly to treatment. Lymphoma in dogs can be classified using the NCI-WF without compromising descriptive accuracy.*[19] Application of the NCI-WF system to tumors is done without regard to immunophenotyping to distinguish B-cells from T-cells. Because immunophenotyping of canine and feline lymphoma is not yet routine and because the NCI-WF provides a pragmatic low/high grading scheme, it is currently recommended for use in dogs and cats.

An updated classification scheme for lymphoid neoplasms known as the Revised European American Lymphoma (REAL) System has been proposed, but it is not in general use for domestic animals.[18] The REAL system combines morphology, immunophenotype, and genotype to categorize lymphoid tumors. The REAL system lists lesions with regard to their histogenic derivation and biological behavior, but without the low- and high-grade separation that is a feature of the NCI-WF.[18]

The American College of Veterinary Pathologists has established a working group to examine and adapt the current (2001) World Health Organization (WHO) classification scheme that is recommended for human lymphoid tumors. The WHO system considers the clinical presentation and disease progression together with the immunophenotype, anatomic site, morphology, and cytogenetics for classifying lymphoid tumors. In the future, histopathology reports and clinical studies may incorporate the WHO classification system. However, until there is general adoption of the WHO system in veterinary medicine, the author prefers to use the NCI-WF (Figures 2, 3, 4, 5, 6, and 7A and B).

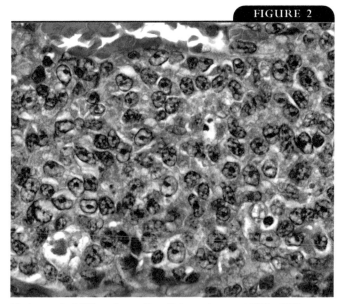

FIGURE 2

High-grade (diffuse large B-cell) Lymphoma, H&E x 800.
Lymph node of a 5 1/2 year old Australian shepherd dog
showing normal lymph node architecture that is replaced by
a diffuse population of lymphocytes that are about 1 1/2 red
cells in diameter. These cells have hyperchromatic chromatin
pattern staining that is more intense at the periphery of the
nuclear membrane. Most cells have a single prominent
nucleolus. The cytoplasm is abundant and highly
amphophilic (variable staining). There are numerous cells
undergoing apoptosis as evident by the tingible body
macrophages (specialized macrophages that phagocytize
lymphocytes that have died by apoptosis) in the lower left
center and right and upper center parts of the image. A
high apoptotic rate is usually accompanied by a high cell
proliferative rate. (Courtesy of Dr. Ted Valli.)

FIGURE 3

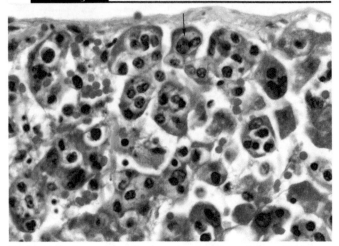

High-grade (large granular lymphocyte) Lymphoma, H&E x 800. Liver from a 10 year old castrated male domestic short haired cat that had icterus, anorexia, and anemia. The normal hepatic parenchyma is heavily colonized with mononuclear cells, 1 to 2 red cells in diameter, with densely staining nuclei. The cells have moderate volumes of cyto-plasm and contain eosinophilic cytoplasmic granules (arrow at top). (Courtesy of Drs. A.J. Johnson and Ted Valli.)

FIGURE 4

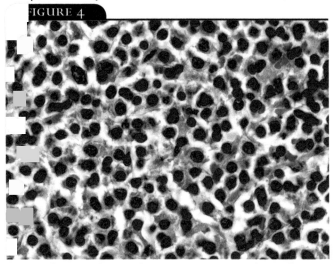

Intermediate-grade Lymphoma, H&E x 800. Spleen of an 11 year old Labrador retriever dog that contained a mass lesion. Cytologically the neoplastic cells have nuclei that are small and lack prominent nucleoli. The cytoplasm is moderate in volume and highly amphophilic. Mitoses are rarely observed. (Courtesy of Dr. Ted Valli.)

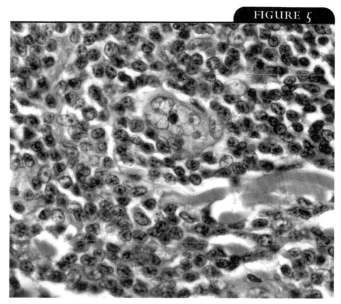

FIGURE 5

Intermediate-grade Lymphoma, H&E x 800. Skin of a 17 year old, castrated male domestic long haired cat that had chronic sub-ungual swelling. The initial biopsy indicated chronic inflammation, but two years later swelling returned to the same area and the digit was removed. The skin is solidly infiltrated with small cell lymphoma that is widely separating the collagen bundles of the dermis. Cytologicially, the neoplastic cells have round to oval nuclei, 1 1/2 to 2 red cells in diameter. The cells have a finely distributed hyperchromatic chromatin pattern with irregular parachromatin clearing in larger cells. Cytoplasm is relatively abundant, characteristically eccentrically distributed and highly amphophilic. Mitoses are rarely observed. (Courtesy of Dr. Ted Valli.)

FIGURE 6

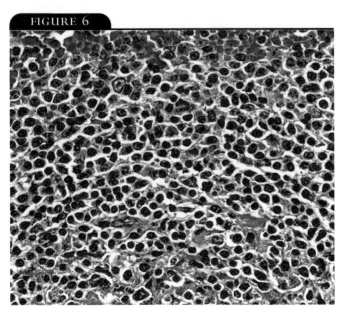

Low-grade lymphoma, H&E x 560. Spleen of a 7 year old spayed female springer spaniel dog that had thrombocytopenia and a splenic mass. Architecturally the mass consists of multi-focal areas of lymphoid proliferation centered on fading germinal centers (bottom) surrounded by homogeneous band of intermediate sized cells. Cytologically, the neoplastic lymphocytes have round nuclei that are approximately 1 1/2 red cells in diameter. Chromatin is at the periphery of the nucleus and most cells have a single prominent central nucleolus. A characteristic feature of these lesions is the abundant cytoplasm that results in relatively uniform spacing of nuclei. Mitoses are characteristically absent. (Courtesy of Dr. Ted Valli.)

FIGURE 7A

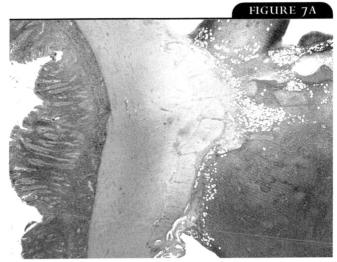

Low-grade Lymphoma, H&E x 170. The small intestine of a mature cat that presented for weight loss with reduced activity and appetite. Hepatosplenomegaly and thickened bowel was found at physical examination. There is a very heavy lymphocytic colonization of the mucosa and submucosa with focal involvement of the mesentary and relative complete sparing of the tunica muscularis. This image indicates the "mucosal homing" that is observed with mucosa associated lymphoid tissue (MALT lymphoma). (Courtesy of Dr. Ted Valli.)

FIGURE 7B

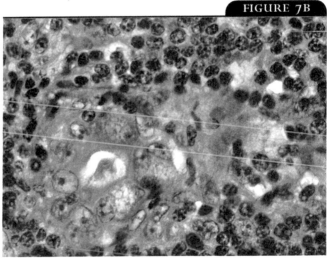

Low-grade Lymphoma, H&E x 800. The same lesion as described in figure 7A at higher magnification. Mitoses are characteristically absent in low-grade lymphoma. (Courtesy of Dr. Ted Valli.)

DOG

One large, multicenter study using the NCI-WF system to evaluate tumors from 285 dogs found that 189 (66.3%) were high-grade tumors, 81 (28.4%) were intermediate-grade tumors, and 15 (5.3%) were low-grade tumors.[20] Dogs with high-grade tumors have been shown to have a poorer prognosis than dogs with low-grade tumors.[21,22]

CAT

A similar study using the NCI-WF system to evaluate 602 cases of feline lymphoma found that 323 (54%) were high-grade, 210 (35%) were intermediate-grade, and 69 (11%) were low-grade tumors.[19]

Immunophenotyping

Immunophenotyping refers to the use of monoclonal antibodies specific for differentiation antigens that are expressed by lymphocytes and accessory immune cells to identify their lineages. Immunophenotyping is an objective complement to conventional assessment of lymphoma that is based solely on morphology. Immunophenotyping can be performed on a variety of specimens, but it is usually performed on unfixed air-dried blood smears, cytological preparations, and fresh tissue that have been snap frozen and sectioned. However, a few mAb have been developed that allow detection of cellular antigens in formalin fixed tissues. Panels of different monoclonal antibiodes (mAb) are applied to the specimens to be examined, and the resultant patterns of expression allow for identification and classification of different cells (T and/or B lymphocytes). This approach has lead to a common nomenclature for antigen expression by a species that are known as "Cluster of Differentiation" antigens or CD antigens depending on how the cells stain with antibody. Far fewer mAb are available that are specific for dogs and cats than are available for humans and mice, but nevertheless, panels of reagents are available that allow T or B cell characterization of lymphoma in dogs and cats (see Figure 5). See Table 2 for additional information on mAb detection of CD antigen expression for cell phenotype identification.

TABLE 2

EXAMPLES OF CLUSTER DIFFERENTIATION (CD) ANTIGEN EXPRESSION FOR LYMPHOCYTE IDENTIFICATION

If Positive	Interpretation
CD1	Expressed by cortical thymocytes, but not by mature T cells. CD1 is useful in identifying histiocytic proliferations
CD3	Expressed only on the surface of mature T cells and thymocytes
CD79a	Expressed by B lymphocytes
CD4	Expressed by T helper cells
CD8	Usually expressed by T cytotoxic cells and some natural killer (NK) cells
CD21	Expressed by mature B cells
CD45	One isoform known as CD45RA is expressed by all B cells and is detectable in formalin fixed tissues
CD34	Expressed by stem and progenitor cells of lymphocytes and other cells. It may be expressed in acute leukemias, but it is usually not expressed in lymphoma that is a malignancy of more mature cells.
BLA.36	Expressed by B lymphocytes

Although at present immunophenotyping is not a standard part of the evaluation of canine and feline lymphoma, it offers the clinician additional information that can be useful in treatment decisions and in estimating prognosis. Immunophenotyping of dog and cat lymphocytes is accomplished with standard immunohistochemical techniques that involve using antibodies against specific surface antigens on lymphocytes that distinguish between B-cell and T-cell tumors. The immunophenotype of lymphoma may have considerable prognostic significance.[19,23-26] If a clinician determines the immunophenotype of a patient's lymphoma, that information should be used to guide treatment choices. For example, because T-cell lymphomas have a poorer prognosis, an aggressive protocol should be used.

A departure from the characterization of lymphoma as either T-cell or B-cell type is found with a variant known as T-cell rich B-cell lymphoma (see Figures 8A and B).[27-29] T-cell rich B-cell lymphoma has been described in both dogs and cats and it is a variant of the diffuse B-cell lymphoma group. It is composed of a mixed cell population of large (lymphoblastic) B-cells that are found within a large background population of small nonneoplastic T-lymphocytes. The neoplastic B-cells typically contribute only 5-25% of the total cell population. This type of lymphoma has been described as a potential "diagnostic pitfall" because the small numbers of neoplastic B-cells in a T-cell rich background makes morphologic diagnosis difficult.[28] The diagnosis of B-cell rich B-cell lymphoma requires both morphologic and immunohistochemical examination of the tumor tissue.[27-29] The significance of this characterization of lymphoma is that it is unique among the presentations previously described in animals. It is also resembles what is known as "human nodular lymphocyte predominance lymphocytic and histiocytic Hodgkin's disease" (NLPHD). NLPHD occurs most commonly in 30-40 year old males that often begins as an isolated adenopathy of months to multi-year duration. The location in affected humans is often is the

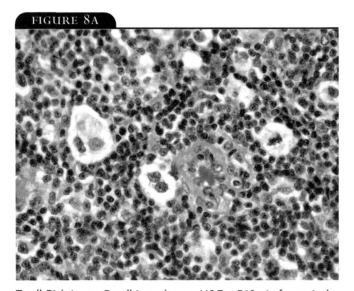

FIGURE 8A

T-cell Rich Large B-cell Lymphoma, H&E x 560. Left cervical lymph node of a 9 year old, spayed female, domestic short-haired cat treated by total surgical excision. The cat had multiple local recurrences that were also excised and was euthanized 3 1/2 yrs later with respiratory difficulty that was caused by widespread necrosis and swelling of the mediastinum. This lymphoma consists of scattered, large, atypical cells with abundant cytoplasm that are often binucleated that are surrounded by closely-packed masses of small benign T-lymphocytes resulting in marked and irregular nodal enlargement. (Courtesy of Dr. Ted Valli.)

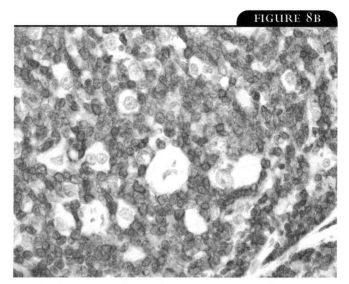

FIGURE 8B

T-cell Rich Large B-cell Lymphoma, CD3 x 560. The same tumor as shown in figure 8A, but showing positive staining for CD3 antigen expression. Note that with specific staining for T-lymphocytes the background population of small lymphocytes is uniformly and heavily labeled with complete sparing of the large non-T lymphocytes that have more abundant cytoplasm. (Courtesy of Dr. Ted Valli.)

cervical, axillary, or inguinal lymph nodes. After treatment, single or multiple relapses often happen at the original site. This behavior is very similar to what has been reported in dogs and cats.[29]

DOG

In several studies in dogs, immunophenotyping has been shown to be an important prognostic marker for overall survival time.[23-26] In a study of immunophenotyping of 58 canine lymphoma biopsy samples, 41 (71%) were determined to be B-cell origin, 14 (24%) were determined to be T-cell origin, and 3 (5%) could not be classified as either B or T types (non-B/non-T cell type). In this study, dogs with a B-cell type of lymphoma had a distinct survival advantage over dogs with T-cell type tumors.[22]

In another study, 36 dogs had B-cell type tumors and 10 had T-cell type. In this study, dogs with B-cell lymphoma had an estimated probability of survival of approximately 45% at one year and 25% at two years, while none of the dogs with T-cell tumors had an esti-mated survival of even a full year.[26]

In a further report of 175 immunophenotyped canine lymphoma biopsy samples, 134 (76%) were determined to be B-cell types and 38 (22%) were determined to be T-cell tumors. For all dogs that achieved a complete remission, the T-cell phenotype was signifi-cantly associated with an early treatment failure.[24]

T-cell lymphomas are often determined to be low or intermediate-grade tumors, but because of their poor prognosis, it has been suggested that all T-cell origin lymphoma in dogs is classified as high-grade clinically regardless of their morphologic features.[22]

A canine example of T-cell rich B-cell lymphoma of the obit that progressed to B-cell lymphoma has been reported.[27] This tumor was composed of predominantely BLA.36 positive large neoplastic lymphoid cells (B-cells) that were mixed with CD3 and CD79a posi-tive small lymphocytes (T-cells). The dog was euthanized approxi-mately 6 months after the start of chemotherapy because of declining health and gastrointestinal and liver involvement.[27]

CAT

Information on immunophenotyping of cat lymphomas is less avail-able than for dogs at this time. In one small study of feline nonep-itheliotrophic lymphoma specimens, 5 of 6 were CD3[+] which means that they were of the T-cell type.[24] However, based on histologic appearance it appears that in cats, the vast majority of cases are B-cell lymphoma. Only 2.1% of 602 cases of feline lymphoma in one study were classified as T-cell origin, while the other 97.9 percent of the cases were classified as some form of B-cell lymphoma.[18]

T-cell rich B-cell lymphoma has also been reported in cats.[28,29] In one case the lymphoma was initially confined to the region of the left parotid salivary gland and it was treated with surgical excision.[28] In another report of eight cases, each tumor was confined to a mass in the neck.[29] In all cases the cats were either FeLV test negative or were not tested during the course of their disease.[28,29] The cats in this study ranged from 4–18 years of age and both sexes were represented in equal numbers. Follow-up was not good in this study, but one cat had two recurrences at 6-month intervals.[29]

AgNOR Assessment

One indicator of tumor proliferation that has been used to predict tumor responsiveness and prognosis is AgNOR enumeration (Figure 9).[30-34] Nucleolar organizer regions (NORs) are loops of DNA that occur in the nucleoli of cells and possess ribosomal RNA genes. The number of NORs reflects the proliferative activity of the cell. The higher the number of NORs observed, the greater the cell's proliferative activity. Silver staining (agryrophilia) and light microscopic evaluation of lymphoma specimens will allow visualization of the NOR's as nuclear dots called AGNORs. The prognostic value of AgNORs has been investigated in several feline and canine tumor types including lymphoma.

The AgNOR frequency per tumor cell nucleus can be determined by averaging the AgNOR count in 100 cells from representative areas of a tumor when viewed by light microscopy under oil immersion (1000X). Although of potential prognostic potential in dogs, AgNOR frequency is rarely determined in clinical cases.

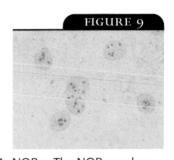

FIGURE 9

Lymphocytes Stained for AgNORs. The NORs are loop aggregates of DNA that occur in the nuclei of cells and they possess rRNA genes (they are sites of RNA transcription). They can be seen with the light microscope as dark dots using a sliver stain reaction (agrophylic) that selectively stains the acidic proteins of the NORs (AgNORs). (Courtesy of Dr. Rose Raskin°.)

DOG

In one study of 55 dogs with lymphoma, AgNOR frequency was determined to correlate with prognosis. The minimum AgNOR frequency was 1.6 and the maximum was 8.2. The mean and median number of AgNORs per cell was 3.7 and 3.5 respectively. The median survival time was 245 days for dogs with tumors with an AgNOR frequency lower than the median value and 486 days for dogs with tumors having an AgNOR frequency above or equal to the median value.[31]

CAT

In a small study of cats with intestinal lymphoma, no association was found between the AgNOR frequency and remission rate, remission duration, or survival.[30]

Clinical Features

Lymphoma in dogs and cats is often classified by anatomic distribution in a patient in addition to histologic grade. The five general anatomic classifications of lymphoma are multicentric, alimentary, mediastinal, extranodal and cutaneous.[35,36] Cutaneous lymphoma is included in the extranodal group by some authors and is addressed in part II of this book.

Multicentric lymphoma is characterized by involvement of multiple lymph nodes usually (but not always) on both sides of the diaphragm. Hepatomegaly, splenomegaly, bone marrow infiltrations and other extranodal involvement may or may not be present.

Alimentary lymphoma in dogs and cats may be characterized by the presence of a solitary mass, multiple masses with or without regional intra-abdominal lymph node involvement, or as a diffusely infiltrating disease of one or more parts of the bowel. Radiographs and ultrasound evaluations of patients with alimentary lymphoma may show focal or diffuse thickening of the gastrointestinal tract, loss of laminations on ultrasound of the stomach or gut wall, regional (mesenteric and iliac) lymphadenomegaly, hepatomegaly and or splenogmegaly. Some patients will have malabsorption and protein loosing enteropathy as a result of their disease and will be malnourished and hypoproteinemic.

The mediastinal form of lymphoma in both dogs and cats usually involves the cranial mediastinal lymph nodes rather than the thymus. Malignant pleural effusion is common and contributes to associated clinical signs of dyspenea, tachypenea, cough, regurgitation, exercise intolerance, dysphagia, and anorexia. Compression of the anterior vena cava may produce generalized cervical and facial edema.

Extranodal lymphoma includes other localizations such as renal, neural, ocular, cardiac, and mucocutaneous (some authors include cutaneous lymphoma with other extranodal locations). Clinical signs may be non-specific, or they may be directly referable to the organ system involved. Regional lymph nodes may or may not be involved in addition to the extranodal localization.

DOG

Up to 84% of cases of lymphoma in dogs will be multicentric in distribution. Alimentary lymphoma is the second most common form (≤ 7%), followed by extranodal (≤ 7%), and mediastinal (≤ 2%).[2,36-41] There are no good data available on the rate of occurrence of cutaneous lymphoma, but it is rare.

Dogs with multicentric disease are usually middle-aged and present with painless, recently noticed lymphadenomegaly of one or more peripheral lymph nodes. Abdominal distension may be secondary to hepatomegaly and/or splenomegaly. Nonspecific signs can include fever, lethargy, anorexia, vomiting and weight loss. Hypercalcemia has been reported in 10-20% of dogs with multicentric lymphoma.[39-41]

Dogs with alimentary lymphoma usually have clinical signs referable to the gastrointestinal system. Vomiting, diarrhea, melena, anorexia, and weight loss are common complaints.[34,36] Dogs usually have a solitary mass associated with the bowel or diffuse disease with or without mesenteric lymph node, spleen, or liver involvement.[36,38]

Up to 40% of dogs with mediastinal lymphoma will be hypercalcemic.[42] Because of the role that calcium ion plays in normal physiology, hypercalcemia can lead to polyuria, polydipsia, vomiting, diarrhea, anorexia, constipation, depression, physical weakness, and cardiac arrhythmias.[21,37,38]

Intravascular lymphoma (malignant angioendotheliomatosis) is a rare angiotopic large-cell lymphoma in which malignant lymphocytes proliferate within lumina of blood vessels in the absence of primary extravascular localization, bone marrow, or leukemia. The dominant clinical signs in 17 dogs with intravascular lymphoma consisted of spinal cord ataxia (n=7), posterior paralysis (n=1), seizures (n=4), and vestibular disease (n=3). Gross lesions were uncommon. Histologically, malignant lymphocytes were most often observed in small to large vessels (usually veins) with thrombus formation and neural malacia. However migration of malignant cells out of blood vessels into the surrounding parenchyma was not observed. In contrast to human cases of intravascular lymphoma where almost all cases are B cell lymphoma, the dogs in this study were both B cell (n=1), T cell (n=8), and non-T, non-B cell (n=6).[44]

A new variant of lymphoma in the dog has been described that is referred to as hepatosplenic lymphoma. One might assume from the name "hepatosplenic" that it is not a new presentation because of the frequency that lymphoma involves the liver and spleen. However, the one veterinary case report of hepatosplenic lymphoma found a dog to have similar specific criteria that have been established for humans with a disorder of the same name. Hepatosplenic lymphoma is characterized by infiltration of the liver, spleen, and bone marrow with neoplastic lymphocytes that express the $\gamma\delta$ T-cell receptor, absence of peripheral lymphadenomegaly, and an aggressive clinical course. The dog in this case report de-compensated quickly and was euthanized.[44a]

CAT

Like dogs, cats with multicentric lymphoma usually have painless, recently noticed lymphadenomegaly of one or more peripheral lymph nodes. Hepatosplenomegaly and bone marrow involvement tend to be secondary and to occur late in the disease process. The multicentric form is most common in younger cats and may be accompanied by a variety of non-specific clinical signs such as anorexia, weight loss, and lethargy. Most cats will test positive for FeLV and concurrent non-regenerative anemia is common.[42,44] Unlike dogs, cats with multicentric lymphoma very rarely have hypercalcemia.

In a retrospective study of hypercalcemia in cats, 21/71 cats had neoplasia while 18/71 had renal failure. Lymphoma and squamous cell carcinoma were the most frequently diagnosed tumors in this study.[45]

The gut is probably the most common site of primary involvement in cats with lymphoma.[46] Cats with alimentary lymphoma tend to be older than 7 years, FeLV test negative (70%), and not anemic. The low rate of FeLV detection is hypothesized to be secondary to these tumors arising from B-cells in the gut-associated lymphoid tissue (GALT). The most common sites of alimentary involvement in decreasing frequency are the small intestines (50%), stomach (25%), ileocecocolic junction, and colon. Cats with alimentary lymphoma characteristically have clinical signs that include weight loss, vomiting, diarrhea, anorexia, and melena. Some patients will have malabsorption and protein loosing enteropathy as a result of their disease and will be malnourished and hypoproteinemic.

Distinguishing between inflammatory bowel disease and lymphoma can be a challenge for the clinician, and at times, the pathologist (Figure 10A and B). There has been considerable speculation that in some cases chronic inflammatory bowel disease in cats may be an antecedent event to lymphoma.[46-50] The presumed relationship between alimentary lymphoma and inflammatory bowel disease is very interesting and perplexing. Although approximately 90% of lymphoma in cats are classified as intermediate or high-grade, two recent studies of gastrointestinal lymphoma in cats suggest that most cases of alimentary lymphoma is due to involvement with small, non-lymphoblastic lymphocytes that might not easily be recognized as malignant.[46,49]

In one of theses studies, 50/67 cats had lymphocytic versus lymphoblastic lymphoma with characteristics of epitheliotrophism. The term "epitheliotrophic" in alimentary lymphoma refers to the

FIGURE 10A

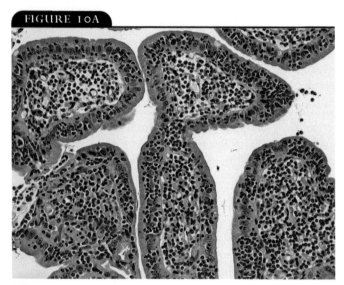

Inflammatory Bowel Disease, H&E x 260. Duodenum of a 15 year old castrated male Maine coon cat that presented for chronic diarrhea and weight loss. Endoscopically obtained biopsies of the mucosal villi demonstrate intense small lymphocytic infiltration into the epithelium and lamina propria. Lesions such as this that persist may be an antecedent event to lymphoma and/or confused with low-grade lymphoma. (Courtesy of Dr. Ted Valli.)

FIGURE 10B

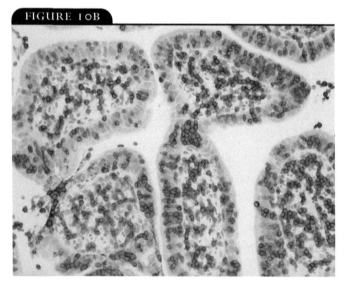

Inflammatory Bowel Disease, CD3 x 260. The same lesion as shown in figure 10A, but showing strong, positive CD3 expression of T-lymphocytes. (Courtesy of Dr. Ted Valli.)

homing of malignant T-lymphocytes to the mucosal epithelium of the intestinal tract that is characteristic of this disorder. The clinical signs and histologic findings in epitheliotrophic alimentary lymphoma will vary widely. Very mild cases may be limited to small numbers of intramucosal small T-cell infiltrates, or extensive remodeling and replacement of normal intestinal architecture by pleomorphic large or anaplastic T-cells.[49]

In the other report of epithelioptrophic lymphoma, 8/10 cats had involvement with small, but malignant lymphocytes, and the other 2/10 cats had involvement with intermediate sized malignant lymphocytes. Immunophenotyping of the cats in this study showed that all 10 cats had T-cell disease. This suggests that on the basis of morphology alone without the ability to perform clonal analysis, it may be extremely difficult to distinguish inflammatory bowel disease (small lymphocytes infiltrating the bowel) from epitheliotrophic lymphoma. In addition, one of the cats in this study had concurrent lymphocytic-plasmacytic gastritis, another cat had concurrent lymphangectasia, and 2 cats had concurrent colitis. Half of the cats in this study had chronic clinical signs of vomiting, diarrhea, decreased appetite, or weight loss persisting for 6 months or longer. In contrast to cats with inflammatory bowel disease that tends to be intermittent, clinical signs in the 10 cats of this study were progressive. There is a hypothesis that feline lymphocytic-plasmacytic inflammatory bowel disease actually represents low-grade intraepitielial T-cell lymphoma and not reactive T-cell proliferation. Six of the 10 cats in this study were treated with chemotherapy. Of the 9 cats that were available for follow-up in this study, 1 cat survived 11 months and 4 cats survived for > 23 months.[46]

A distinct subpopulation of cats with lymphoma has been described in which the tumors are composed of large granular lymphocytes (LGL) (Figure 11).[51] These large granular lymphocytes are a morphologically distinct population of lymphocytes characterized by abundant cytoplasm and prominent azurophilic granules.[51] Natural killer cells and cytotoxic T lymphocytes are examples of LGL's.[51,52] The majority of these tumors originate in the gut, especially the jejunum and mesenteric lymph nodes and an abdominal mass is usually easily palpated. Clinical presentation includes anorexia, lethargy, vomiting and/or diarrhea. Laboratory abnormalities can

FIGURE 11

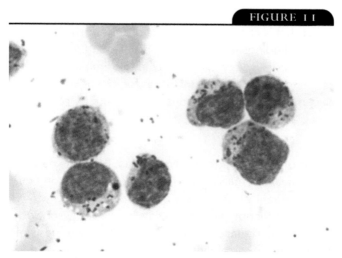

Large Granular Lymphocytes in Peripheral Blood from a Cat. Note the large azurophilic granules. (Courtesy of Dr. Rose Raskin©.)

include leukocytosis, hypoalbuminemia, hypocalcemia, increased AST activity, and increased concentrations of serum bilirubin. In one study, all cats with this type of lymphoma were FeLV test negative.[53] In a different study of large granular lymphocyte lymphoma in 6 cats, 3 cats had the main involvement localized to the gastrointestinal tract and jejunal lymph nodes, but 3 had wide spread organ involvement to locations such as the lung, myocardium, precardiac mediastinum, salivary gland and spinal cord. In addition, leukemia was present in two of the cats.[52]

Cats with mediastinal lymphoma tend to be between 2 and 3 years of age and to test positive for FeLV (Figure 12A, B, C and D). This form of lymphoma in cats usually involves the cranial and caudal mediastinal lymph nodes, rather than the thymus gland. Pleural effusion containing malignant lymphocytes contributes to the clinical signs of dyspnea, coughing, and exercise intolerance. Entrapment and compression of the esophagus by the mediastinal tumor will often result in dysphagia, regurgitation, and anorexia. The thorax may be non-compressible during the physical examination. Hypercalcemia is rare.[54]

Clinical signs of lymphoma of the nasal and/or paranasal sinuses include dyspnea, nasal discharge, facial distortion, and anorexia. One study concluded that FeLV test positive cats with nasal/paranasal sinus lymphoma were more likely to develop

FIGURE 12A

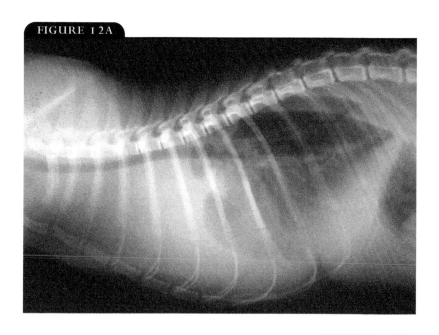

A. Lateral radiograph of a cat with mediastinal lymphoma. Note the free fluid in the pleural space (Figures 12C-D). Palpation of this cat's thorax would be characterized as "non-compressible."

B. VD radiograph of a cat with mediastinal lymphoma. Note the wide mediastinum and the displacement of the trachea to the cat's left.

FIGURE 12B

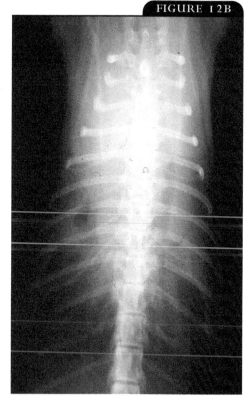

FIGURE 12C

FIGURE 12D

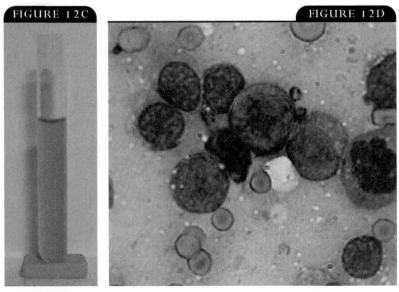

C. Mediastinal fluid associated with mediastinal mass
D. Cytology of fluid from pleural space of cat in figures 12A and B. Note the large lymphocytes (blasts) and mititoc figures.

systemic disease and recommended systemic chemotherapy instead of local therapy such as radiation therapy.[55]

Renal lymphoma is the most common neoplasm affecting the kidneys in cats (Figures 13A and B).[56,57] It can occur as the primary tumor or in association with an alimentary or multicentric distribution. One study reported that the mean age of 28 cats with renal lymphoma was 7 years and that 50% of the cats tested positive for FeLV.[57] Presenting signs are non-specific (anorexia, lethargic, vomiting) and are due to renal dysfunction or significant tumor size. Abdominal palpation reveals unilateral or bilateral renomegaly, often with irregular surface contours. Many cats with renal lymphoma are also anemic.[56,57] A biochemistry profile can help detect azotemia and hyperphosphatemia. Urine specific gravity may be isosthenuric. Central nervous system metastasis was reported in 40% of the cats with renal lymphoma.[57]

Primary or secondary ocular lymphoma occurs in about 10% of cases.[1,58] Lymphoma behind the eye can create buphthalmous. The third eyelid and palpebral conjunctiva may be infiltrated and bulge through the palpebral fissure. Intraocular involvement is relatively common and is frequently manifested by anterior uveal and chorioretinal abnormalities.[58] Because ocular and orbital lymphoma can occur secondary to FeLV infection, the FeLV status of cats with ocular inflammation with or without obvious tumor formation should be determined.[59]

Unusual manifestations of lymphoma in cats are occasionally encountered. Hypoadrenocorticism as the primary manifestation of lymphoma in two cats was recently reported.[60] Although most cats with naturally occurring hypoadrenocorticism have idiopathic adrenal atrophy, these two cats had lymphoma infiltrating their adrenal glands and had typical signs of adrenal insufficiency like lethargy, weight loss, weakness, hyperkalemia, hyponatremia,

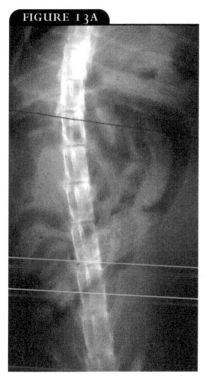
FIGURE 13A

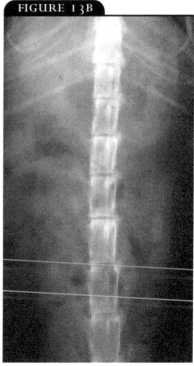
FIGURE 13B

A. Lateral Radiograph of Cat with Renal Lymphoma. Note the enlarged, irregular kidneys.
B. VD radiograph of the same cat in figure 13A five months after receiving chemotherapy for lymphoma. Note the decrease in size and the return to normal renal contours. This cat also experienced a return to normal renal function as determined by clinical laboratory analysis.

azotemia, and flat ACTH response tests. Both of these individuals were euthanized within a short time of their diagnosis.[60]

Clinical Laboratory Findings

A variety of clinical laboratory abnormalities are encountered in dogs and cats with lymphoma. Routine laboratory testing will usually define most problems, although special investigations such as bone marrow cytology may be needed for complete assessment.

DOG

Anemia is one of the most common laboratory abnormalities associated with lymphoma in dogs, and it is reported to occur in up to 38% of cases.[61] The anemia is most often described as a normochromic, normocytic, non-regenerative 'anemia of chronic disease' wherein a clear cause of the anemia is not found.[62] Anemia of this kind may be secondary to chronic inflammation associated with the disease, decreased RBC survival time, abnormal iron metabolism, or decreased bone marrow response to erythropoietin. The persistent use of cytotoxic chemotherapeutic drugs may perpetuate the nonregenerative state.[37] Immune-mediated hemolytic anemia, with or without thrombocytopenia, may also be present.[37] The primary complaint of the owner may be referable to the anemia (weakness, pale mucous membranes). Anemic dogs with lymphoma may be positive for ANA, Coombs' or platelet Factor III, but these findings have few clinical consequences beyond the impact from anemia.[37]

Thrombocytopenia is reported to occur in up to 58% of dogs with lymphoproliferative disease.[61,63] Decreased platelet numbers are usually due to decreased platelet production secondary to direct invasion of bone marrow (myelophthisis) and a diminished capacity of bone marrow to produce megakaryocytes.[61,63] Other mechanisms causing a decline in platelets include sequestration, immune-mediated destruction, and increased consumption.[63]

Variations from normal in total leukocyte counts commonly occur in dogs with lymphoma. In a study of 24 dogs with lymphoma, leukopenia occurred in 19% and leukocytosis occurred in 32%.[21]

Lymphocytosis and lymphopenia in dogs in the same study occurred with similar frequency (20% and 25%, respectively).[21] Infiltration of the bone marrow has been variably reported (rare to 50%), likely reflecting inconsistencies of bone marrow evaluation among different published studies.[62] Most publications do not specifically report having evaluated the bone marrow, and the results also vary with the diagnostic sampling method(s) used.[63]

Hypercalcemia is a relatively common paraneoplastic syndrome associated with canine lymphoma. It has been reported in 10-40% of dogs with this tumor (see section on paraneoplastic syndromes for additional information on hypercalcemia).[1,21]

CAT

Anemia is also a common finding in cats with lymphoma, especially among those that test positive for FeLV.[42,63] Hardy reported that 68% of FeLV test positive cats with lymphoma have anemia, while < 10% of the FeLV test negative lymphoma cats are anemic.[66] The anemia is most often normochromic, normocytic, or nonregenerative 'anemia of chronic disease' where a clear cause of the anemia is not found.[42,67] As with dogs, this type of anemia may be due to chronic inflammation associated with the disease, decreased RBC lifespan, abnormal iron metabolism, decreased bone marrow response, or decreased iron stores. FeLV infection may also affect the bone marrow more directly and cause myelodysplastic diseases and red cell aplasia.[42] Immune-mediated hemolytic anemia, with or without thrombocytopenia, can also be present.

Thrombocytopenia is less commonly observed in cats with lympho-proliferative disease than in dogs.[64] Decreased platelet numbers may occur secondary to decreased platelet production from myelo-phythesis.[64] Other mechanisms causing platelet numbers to decline include sequestration, immune-mediated destruction and increased consumption secondary to disseminated intravascular coagulation.[64] In a retrospective study of 41 cats with thrombocytopenia, 12% were identified as having lymphoproliferative malignancies.[68]

Leukocytosis, especially with lymphocytosis, should lead to critical evaluation of peripheral blood smears by the clinician and a clinical pathologist. Circulating abnormal lymphoid cells indicate bone marrow involvement that in one study suggested a poorer prognosis for remission.[42] Bone marrow aspirates should be performed as part of staging, especially in cats with lymphoma affecting the spinal cord. In a report of 16 cats with spinal lymphoma that had bone marrow aspirates performed, 11 cats (69%) had lymphoblasts in the bone marrow.[69]

While hypercalcemia is a relatively common paraneoplastic syndrome associated with canine lymphoma, it is a rare occurrence in cats.[21,66] Most cases of hypercalcemia reported in cats have been associated with lymphoproliferative diseases.[50,54] The most common clinical signs associated with hypercalcemia in cats include anorexia, vomiting, weight loss, and dehydration.[54] Hypercalcemia does not seem to cause polydipsia and polyuria in cats as it may in dogs.[54,69]

Monoclonal gammopathy has been described in cats with lymphoma and is primarily due to the increased production of IgG.[62,67,70] Clinical signs are primarily associated with hyperviscosity resulting in ophthalmic, neurologic, hematologic, and renal abnormalities.[62,67,70] Clinical signs in cats with monoclonal gammopathy can also be non-specific and include anorexia and lethargy.[70] Protein electrophoresis and immunoelectrophoresis help establish a diagnosis after the recognition of an abnormally elevated total serum protein concentration. Differential diagnoses for a monoclonal gammopathy in a cat include multiple myeloma, amyloidosis, and benign hyperglobulinemia.[62]

Paraneoplastic Syndromes

HYPERCALCEMIA

Hypercalcemia associated with lymphoma is characterized by persistent elevations of measured total serum calcium concentrations. Hypercalcemia is one of the most common paraneoplastic syndromes in animals, and it is especially common in dogs with lymphoma.[21]

Clinical signs of hypercalcemia are referable to the role that calcium plays in normal physiology in maintaining stability and excitability of neuronal membranes, and in the contractility of smooth, skeletal, and cardiac muscle. Clinical signs of hypercalcemia include mental depression, weakness, anorexia, vomiting, and arrhythmia. Calcium nephropathy and renal failure may occur if the calcium x phosphorus product exceeds 70. Polyuria (from hyposthenuria) with a compensatory polydipsia may be an early sign of hypercalcemia because calcium ion antagonizes antidiuretic hormone effects on the distal nephron and collecting ducts.

Interpretation of serum calcium concentrations should reflecte consideration of blood pH and total protein. Since almost 1/2 of the total serum calcium is non-ionized and bound to albumin, hypoalbuminemia will lower the normal upper limit of serum calcium by relatively increasing the unbound (ionized) form. Acidosis will also disturb the equilibrium between ionized and non-ionized calcium (bound and unbound) in favor of the ionized form. Until recently, correcting total serum calcium based on albumin concentrations and total protein concentrations has been done with the following formulas. The first of these formulas was used most often to help determine if a patient is hypercalcemic relative to the albumin concentration.

$$\text{Corrected serum Ca} = \text{measured Ca} - \text{albumin} + 3.5$$

or

$$\text{Corrected serum Ca} = \text{measured Ca} - (0.4 \times \text{total protein}) + 3.3$$

These calculations are no longer relied on to determine hypercalcemia. Most clinicians now rely on a measuring serum ionized calcium concentration for that determination. Serum ionized calcium concentrations can be determined by most commercial laboratories, and values can be compared to reference ranges for calcium. If there is any question about the potential for hypercalcemia, a serum ionized calcium concentration should be measured.

The treatment of hypercalcemia is always best directed at treatment of the underlying malignancy. Intravenous saline diuresis at 1 to 2 x maintenance needs, sodium wasting diuretics such as furosemide (only in a well hydrated patient), and corticosteroids (prednisone 1 mg/kg bid) can be helpful in the short-term treatment of hypercalcemia while a comprehensive plan for cancer treatment is made and agreed to by the owner. Other treatments advocated in human medicine such as calcitonin or gallium nitrate are either expensive, subject to only brief clinical efficacy, or need evaluation in the veterinary setting before they can be recommended.

However, bisphosphonates such as pamidronate disodium appear to be safe for treating hypercalcemia and are frequently employed in veterinary oncology for that purpose. Bisphosphonates inhibit normal and pathological bone resorption and reduce serum calcium by inhibiting osteoclasts, retarding the deposition of hydroxyapatite in bone collagen, increasing unmineralized osteoid, and inhibiting the formation of calcium phosphate crystals. Pamidronate and diuresis are suggested as primary treatments for human childhood and adult hypercalcemia of malignancy. No definitive doses have been established for dogs or cats, but reported doses for dogs range from .65 to 2.0 mg/kg intravenously. A dose of 1.3 mg/kg in saline intravenously over 2 hours was used effectively in one dog with hypercalcemia secondary to an apocrine gland adenocarcinoma. [70a] Electrolyte abnormalities are recognized complications of bisphosphonate treatment in humans and have been observed in dogs (example; hypomagnesemia). Relief from hypercalcemia in dogs with lymphoma may last for weeks following treatment with bisphosphonates. Hypercalcemia in cats can also be safely treated with pamidronate using the same dose as for dogs.[70a, 70b]

Dog

The most common tumors in dogs to have associated hypercalcemia are lymphoma, adenocarcinoma of the apocrine glands of the anal sac, and multiple myeloma.[1,71] A variety of other tumor types in dogs (mammary gland adenocarcinoma, nasal adenocarcinoma, pulmonary adenocarcinoma, thyroid carcinoma, thymoma, osteosarcoma, and squamous cell carcinoma) have also been described as occasionally associated with hypercalcemia.[71] Some reports describe the incidence of hypercalcemia associated with lymphoma in dogs at up to 40%, and many hypercalcemic dogs with lymphoma have the mediastinal form.

Hypercalcemia associated with lymphoma may be due to humoral hypercalcemia of malignancy, or local resorption of bone induced by lymphoma that has metastasized to the bone marrow. However, most dogs with lymphoma and hypercalcemia have a humoral component since extensive bone resorption may occur distant to the site of tumor metastases in bone.[62]

Local osteolysis may be produced by the direct infiltration and resorption of the bone by osteoclast activating factors produced and released by tumor cells. These substances have, at various times, been identified as interleukins, tumor necrosis factor, lympho-toxin, colony-stimulating factors or interferon γ.[62]

In one study where N-terminal PTH-related protein (PTHrP), N-terminal PTH, and 1, 25 dihydroxyvitamin D concentrations were measured in normal dogs, dogs with cancer associated hypercal-cemia, dogs with "other" tumors, and dogs with parathyroid adenomas, PTHrP was undetectable in normal dogs and increased in hypercalcemic dogs with apocrine gland adenocarcinoma of the anal sac, dogs with lymphoma, and dogs with "other" tumors. The PTHrP concentrations decreased in dogs with lymphoma and anal sac adenocarcinoma after successful treatment. The PTHrP concentration had a significant linear correlation with total serum calcium in dogs with hypercalcemia and anal sac andenocarcinoma or lymphoma. Serum N-terminal PTH concentrations were usually in the normal range for all groups of dogs except for dogs with parathyroid adenoma where they were increased. The serum N terminal PTH concentrations increased after successful treatment. Serum 1,25 dihy-droxyvitamin D concentrations were decreased, normal, or increased in dogs with cancer associated hypercalcemia. However, concentra-tions decreased after successful treatment of the primary tumor. It appears that circulating concentrations of PTHrP are consistently increased in dogs with cancer associated hypercalcemia and PTHrP appears to play an important role in the induction of hypercalcemia.[72]

Cat

Hypercalcemia is rare in cats with cancer, but it has been reported in cats with lymphoma, squamous cell carcinoma, myelosclerosis, myelo-proliferative disease, multiple myeloma, and lymphocytic leukemia.[73,74]

Mechanisms of hypercalcemia in cats with cancer have not been explored. However, in a report of hypercalcemia in two cats with multiple myeloma, the assumption was made that the mechanism involved PTH or PTH-like activity because of the pattern of increased total calcuim and ionized calcium concentrations with decreased plamsa phosphrus concentrations.[74]

MYELOFIBROSIS

Myelofibrosis has been reported in both dogs and cats with lymphoma. Myelofibrosis can be associated with myeloproliferative disorders, secondary to bone marrow damage, distant cancer effects, or it may be of unknown cause. Myelofibrosis is a rare clinical finding in dogs and cats with lymphoma.[71]

EOSINOPHILIA

The concentration of eosinophils is normally tightly regulated and accounts for a small segment of peripheral blood neutrophils. Eosinophilia can be harmful because of the proinflammatory effects of eosinophils, or it may be helpful because of their antiparasitic effects.

Eosinophils are produced in bone marrow for pluripotential stem cells. Interleukin –3, interlukin –5, and granulocyte-macrophage colony stimulating factor (GM-CCSF) are the principal cytokines that govern and regulate eosinophil numbers. Of these, interleukin –5 is the most specific for eosinophils and is responsible for their selective differentiation. Interleukin –5 also stimulates the release of eosinophils from bone marrow into systemic circulation. Overproduction of interleukin –5 in some species can result in a profound eosinophilia. In humans, diseases associated with eosinophilia without expansion of other blood-cell liniages are usually accompanied by an overproduction of interleukin –5. The mechanisms of cytokine overproduction may include a response to T-helper lymphocytes, the activation of a gene transcription due to a chromosome translocation, and/or the malignant expansion of T-cell clones that produce interleukin –5. Eosinophilia is a clinical finding in some humans with lymphoma or gastrointestinal malignancies.[75]

Dog

Profound eosinophilia is rare in dogs with malignant disease. It is more common in dogs with pulmonary eosinophilia secondary to causes such as hypersensitivity to inhaled antigens, severe gastrointestinal parasitism, pulmonary parasites, and heartworm. Profound eosinophilia has been reported in a dog with an oral fibrosarcoma.[76] Eosinophilia is not associated with lymphoma in dogs.

Cat

Profound eosinophila is also rare in cats. However, profound eosinophilia has been reported in a single cat with transitional cell carcinoma of the bladder.[77] Profound eosinophilia in cats is more commonly observed in individuals with what is commonly termed hypereosinophilic syndrome and/or pulmonary eosinophilia.

Hypereosinophilic syndrome is characterized by bone marrow hyperplasia of eosinophilic precursors and multiple organ infiltration by mature eosinophils. Eosinophilic leukemia is a similar disorder (may be a variant of hypereosinophilic syndrome), but the eosinophils involved are less mature.[78] Neither hypereosinophilic syndrome nor eosinophilic leukemia appears to be associated with FeLV infection.

Pulmonary eosinophilia may be seen in cats with hypersensitivity disorders that affect the lung. Pulmonary eosinophilia may be triggered by a variety of inhaled environmental stimulants, lung parasites, migrating larvae, and heartworm.

Absolute eosinophilia has been reported in cats with lymphoma, mast cell tumors, carcinomas, and other sarcomas.[79] However, eosinophilia is not a reliable hallmark of lymphoma in cats.

POLYCYTHEMIA

Polycythemia in ill animals is usually a relative event secondary to dehydration. Absolute polycythemia must be evaluated with an arterial PO_2 concentration. Polycythemia associated with a decreased arterial PO_2 concentration is an appropriate systemic response and is common with disorders such as chronic alveolar hypoventilation, severe and chronic pulmonary disease, cardiac right-to-left shunts, and living at high altitude. Polycythemia associated with normal arterial PO_2 may be due to hormonal stimulation (hyperadrenalcorticism, corticosteroid administration, androgen administration), inappropriate secretion of erythropoietin or erythropoietin-like substances (renal lymphoma, renal carcinoma, renal fibrosarcoma, other tumors, pyelonephritis), or polycythemia vera (a primary myeloproliferative disorder of bone marrow). Polycythemia secondary to erythropoietin or erythropoietin-like substances is rare in dogs and cats with lymphoma.[71]

METABOLIC EPIDERMAL NECROSIS (TOXIC EPIDERMAL NECROLYSIS)

Metabolic epidermal necrosis in dogs is most frequently associated with hepatic disease and glucagon secreting tumors. In cats it has been associated with thymic amyloidosis, pancreatic carcinoma, lymphoma, and in the author's experience, with an IgA secreting multiple myeloma. The footpads and periorbital are usually affected with crusting and necrotic lesions, but this is not a consistent finding.[80]

Symmetric cutaneous necrosis of the hind feet of a cat with multicentric follicular lymphoma was recently reported.[81] The cat was a 7-year-old castrated male domestic shorthair cat and had a history of lethargy and swelling of the hind feet for one month prior to diagnosis. On admission to the referral hospital, the skin of the hind feet from 2 cm proximal to the metatarsophalangeal joints to the phalanges was symmetrically necrotic. The pads and skin were hard and leathery, and necrotic skin was starting to separate from the underlying tissues in the metatarsal region. The cat was able to walk well and did not have signs of pain on palpation of the necrotic skin or feet. Slight mineralization of the digital pads was apparent on radiographs of the feet.

Lymphoma was diagnosed from a fine needle aspirate of the liver. The pancreas had disorganized acinar exocrine cells that were consistent with early nodules of adenocarcinoma. Microscopically, several arterioles in the deep dermis were partially or completely occluded by thrombi. No cause of ischemic necrosis of the skin in this cat could be identified (trauma, frostbite, burns, snake and other bits, vasculitis, hypertrophic cardiomyopathy, cold agglutinin disease, lymphomatoid granulomatosis, etc). Although cutaneous necrosis can develop with pancreatic adenocarcinoma in humans, the regional cutaneous necrosis in this cat was attributed to the lymphoma rather than the pancreatic carcinoma because the lymphoma was more advanced.[81]

Diagnosis and Staging

Diagnosis and staging are important steps in the overall management of dogs and cats with lymphoma. A tentative diagnosis may be suspected from the initial physical examination findings, but definitive diagnosis requires biopsy. A definitive diagnosis may be established after cytologic assessment with a fine needle aspiration biopsy or histologic assessment with a tissue biopsy (needle core biopsy or surgical biopsy). Fine needle aspiration and tissue biopsy procedures should be viewed as complimentary to each other. Although a definitive diagnosis may be established with either, a more accurate and complete characterization of the tumor can only be done with histologic assessment.

The complete patient assessment of dogs and cats with lymphoma require the following: A thorough medical history, complete physical examination, CBC, serum chemistry panel, urinalysis, fine needle aspiration biopsy of a lesion for initial diagnosis, a needle core biopsy or surgical biopsy for confirmation and additional characterization such as phenotyping or AgNOR assay if desired, radiographs of the thorax (three views) and abdomen (2 views), a bone marrow aspiration biopsy, and a complete ophthalmic examination. An abdominal sonogram should be done to peruse abnormalities detected by radiography. Some oncologists prefer to substitute the abdominal sonogram for the abdominal radiographs, but this practice increases the likelihood of mistakes in basic staging because each modality differs in its ability to detect disease. Radiographs are superior to sonograms in defining spatial resolution and organ orientation and making radiographic images is largely independent of operator skill. Sonograms define tissue contrast and invasiveness better than do radiographs, but spatial relationships are not defined as well, and the validity of the scan is highly dependent on operator skill.

This comprehensive approach to patient assessment is necessary to identify all of the medical problems of the patient including any associated paraneoplastic syndromes, to identify any organ system involvement that will effect patient tolerance and response to chemotherapy, and to allow for complete clinical staging of the patient. Any procedure or test omitted for whatever reason has the potential to compromise patient response to treatment and survival. However, when circumstances conspire to preclude a complete evaluation, the staging can be reduced to its clinical essentials and still be adequate for the majority of clinical cases (Table 3).

Dogs and cats can be staged in similar manner (Table 4).[43,79,82] Clinical stages I through V in dogs and cats can be determined from identical criteria, however in recent years there has been a trend among veterinary oncologists to stage cats slightly differently (Tables 4 and 5).[43,79] Cats are sometime referred to by "Mooney

TABLE 3
RECOMMENDED AND ALTERNATE DIAGNOSTIC WORKUPS

Recommended Diagnostic Work-up for Complete Staging	Acceptable Alternative Work-up for Staging
CBC	CBC
Serum biochemistry	Serum biochemistry
Urinalysis	Urinalysis
FeLV (cat only)	FeLV (cat only)
Feline Immunodeficiency virus (FIV) (cat only)	Feline Immunodeficiency virus (FIV) (cat only)
Three view thoracic radiographs	Two view thoracic radiographs
Two view abdominal radiographs	Two view abdominal radiographs
Abdominal sonogram	or abdominal sonogram
Echocardiogram if doxorubicin use anticipated	Echocardiogram if doxorubicin use anticipated
Complete ophthalmological exam	Fine needle aspiration biopsy of lymph node or organ
Fine needle aspiration biopsy of lymph node or organ	Bone marrow aspiration biopsy if circulating malignant lymphocytes present or if any cytopenias present
Trucut or surgical biopsy of lymph node or organ or histologic grading	
Immunophenotyping	
AgNOR evaluation	
Bone marrow aspiration biopsy	
Bone marrow core biopsy	

TABLE 4
CLINICAL STAGING FOR DOGS AND CATS*

Stage I
A single lymph node or anatomic location affected

Stage II
Multiple lymph nodes or anatomic sites affected on one side of
the diaphragm

Stage III
Multiple lymph nodes or anatomic sites affected on both sides of
the diaphragm

Stage IV
Stages I-III with liver and/or spleen involvement

Stage V
Stages I-IV with involvement of the CNS or bone marrow or both

*From Owen LN. TNM classification of tumors of domestic animals. 1st ed. Geneva,
Switzerland: World Health Organization; 1980:46-47.

TABLE 5
CLINICAL STAGING FOR CATS

Stage I
A single tumor (extranodal) or single anatomic area (nodal) includes
primary intrathoracic tumors

Stage II
A single tumor (extranodal) with regional lymph node involvement
Two or more nodal areas on the same side of the diaphragm
Two single (extranodal) tumors with or without regional lymph node
involvement on the same side of the diaphragm
A rescetable primary gastrointestinal tumor, usually in the ileocecal
area, with or without involvement of associated mesenteric nodes only

Stage III
Two single tumors (extranodal) on opposite sides of the diaphragm
Two or more nodal areas above and below the diaphragm
All extensive primary un-resectable intraabdominal disease
All paraspinal or epidural tumors regardless of other tumor site or sites

Stage IV
Stages I-III with liver and/or spleen involvement

Stage V
Stages I-IV with initial involvement of CNS or bone marrow or both

From Mooney SC, Hayes AA. Lymphoma in the cat: an approach to diagnosis and management. Sem in Vet Med Surg (Small Anim) 1986;1:51-57.

Stage" after the primary author of the paper that introduced this method of staging.

Staging of patients is important because it allows for more accurate and meaningful comparisons of treatment response and survival data between published studies, for assisting selection of chemotherapy protocols that are most appropriate for our patients, and for predicting clinical outcome as we interact with and inform owners.

Evaluating Treatment Protocols for Canine and Feline Lymphoma

In almost all cases, the principal treatment modality for dogs and cats with lymphoma will be chemotherapy. There are many chemotherapy treatment protocols available to veterinarians and choosing between them may be difficult. The typical response rate varies from 65% to 96% and a first remission duration of 6 to 9 months is common.[1] Second remissions are usually shorter than the first, and overall survival for most dogs treated with common protocols is between 10 and 12 months. When choosing a protocol, it is important to balance expected benefit (published response data) against toxicity, cost, and convenience for the owner.

When discussing chemotherapy with an owner you may find that they have preconceptions based on their experience with a family member or friend with cancer. Most chemotherapy protocols used to treat canine lymphoma are associated with minimal to moderate toxicity. More aggressive protocols have been used in dogs and published, but these rarely find wide use among practicing veterinarians because most owners are not willing to have their dogs experience a treatment that carries a significant risk for being debilitating or life-threatening.

Owners must understand the difference between palliation and cure and they, together with their veterinarian, must understand that the most reasonable goal for the vast majority of dogs with lymphoma is an extension of a good quality of life and not cure. Palliation for many months is usually an attainable goal, while "cure" is usually not attainable.

It is important to understand the emotional and financial resources of the owner before advising one protocol over another. Some protocols are virtually absent of any side effects that the owner might notice, while others may be associated with mild to severe side effects. Likewise, some protocols can be quite expensive, require careful and expensive monitoring, while others are relatively inexpensive and require no monitoring.

As you evaluate the literature in preparation for selecting a protocol, it is important that you completely understand the common terms associated with reporting results. The following are standard definitions that you should be familiar with.

Complete response (CR) is used to describe complete remission and disappearance of all clinically detectable disease. Partial remission (PR) is used to describe at least a 50% reduction in the clinically detectable tumor burden without the appearance of new lesions. Stable Disease (SD) is used to describe a less than 50% reduction in the overall tumor burden without the appearance of new lesions. Progressive disease (PD) is defined as a greater than 50% increase in tumor burden and/or the detection of new lesions. Different reports of efficacy may define these terms differently. Not all reports of chemotherapy efficacy discriminate between CR and PR. Some authors may lump them together under the term of "response rate." "Response rate" as a term is sometimes used to put protocols in the best light possible because the number of dogs that "respond" will always be higher than the number of dogs in CR or PR alone. Another term that has recently entered the literature is "progression free interval." This usually indicates the time from the onset of remission until relapse and is generally the same as "duration of first remission."

Whatever terms are used in the publications that you use for guidance, they must be defined within the text to be useful for comparisons. For example, unless stated, the duration of first remission could be (and has been) defined as the time from onset of clinical signs until relapse, the time from clinical diagnosis until relapse, the time from biopsy confirmation until relapse, or the time from the start of chemotherapy until relapse. Likewise, overall survival needs clear definition to be useful. Survival can also be determined from various points from first recognition of clinical signs to death on through to the first day of chemotherapy to death. Unless you know how the parameters are defined, a false impression may be created that one protocol is better than another simply because the starting point for determining clinical response is earlier than another.

It is important to understand the difference between the statistical terms *mean* and *median*. Both mean and median are used to describe the central tendency of a set of numbers. Mean and median values may be the same or different. Older literature will often report mean values for some series of numbers relating to response, duration of remission, or survival, etc. The mean value of a set of numbers is the *average* value in the set. It may or may not give you a good indication of the center of the number set (that indicates the average patient response). For example if you take the number set 1, 2, 3, 4, 5, 6, and 7, the mean value would be determined by adding all the numbers (28) and dividing by the number of numbers (7) so the mean value would be 4. In this example the number 4 is a good indication of central tendency (average patient response). However, if you take the number set 1, 2, 3, 4, 5, 6, and 100 you get a mean of 17.28. By including the outlier in the average, you get a false impression of where the center of the number set (average patient response) is. If these number sets related to prognosis or response, is it more likely that your patient's response will be a 4 or a 17.28?

Median values give a clear indication of central tendency in a number set with one or more outliers and can be more valuable to us clinically. Median values are the center number in the number set regardless of how many numbers there are. In the above example of the number set of 1, 2, 3, 4, 5, 6, and 7, the median value is the same as the mean value (4) and both are good indicators of central tendency. In the second example using the number set 1, 2, 3, 4, 5, 6, and 100, the median value is still 4 because it is the center number of the series (when the series of numbers is an even number the middle two numbers are averaged to arrive at the median value). In almost all situations, a median value will have more importance to the clinician than the mean value because it is a better indicator of central tendency and relates better to expected patient responses.

Other terms of importance in the literature are induction chemotherapy, maintenance chemotherapy, adjuvant chemotherapy, and neoadjuvant chemotherapy. Induction chemotherapy is that therapy used to induce a remission. It typically is relatively aggressive when compared to the maintenance phase and is intended to quickly induce a remission. Induction chemotherapy is also occasionally used to denote chemotherapy for a patient with advanced disease and for whom there is no effective advanced treatment. Maintenance chemotherapy is used in some protocols after induction to "maintain" remission. It is typically less aggressive than induction and is usually associated with fewer side effects. Adjuvant chemotherapy is a term used to denote when chemotherapy is given *after* a different primary treatment such as surgery or radiation therapy is used. Neoadjuvant chemotherapy is a term that is used to denote chemotherapy given at the earliest possible time in the overall treatment plan for a patient. Depending on the circumstances, this could mean chemotherapy given during or immediately after some loco-regional therapy such as surgery or radiation therapy.

PERFORMANCE AND TOXICITY ASSESSMENT

Patients in many clinical studies are evaluated using an objective/subjective performance scale so that differences in clinical status prior to and after treatment can be assessed. Performance assessment of patients prior to entering, during, and after entering clinical trials also allows for patients to be categorized into similar groups based on clinical condition at any point in the disease process rather than making comparisons between groups of patients that includes asymptotic and critically ill. A commonly used measure of performance status in veterinary medicine is a modified Karnofsky scale (Table 6). Performance assessment is not routinely made on all patients, but extra information can be gathered from studies where the effects of performance status on treatment outcome or the effects of treatment on patient performance (treat-

TABLE 6
MODIFIED KARNOFSKY PERFORMANCE SCALE

General Category	Index	Specific Criteria
Normal activity	0	Able to perform at pre-disease level.
Restricted activity	1	Decreased activity from pre-disease level, but able to function as an acceptable pet.
Compromised activity	2	Ambulatory only to the point of eating, sleeping, and consistently defecating and urinating in acceptable areas.
Disabled	3	Requires enteral or parenteral nutrition. Unable to confine urination and defecation to acceptable areas.
Dead	4	Dead

ment morbidity) have been included. More recent publications are beginning to reference performance assessment in their results.

Some reports of chemotherapy will have clear references to toxicity, and some will actually score hematologic and gastrointestinal toxicity. There are no standardized toxicity scores for use in veterinary medicine, but several have been adopted from human medicine. It is important to closely inspect toxicity when evaluating a protocol. Table 7 illustrates one useful toxicity grading scheme that is applicable to dogs and cats.[83]

n=?

The n of a study is usually the number of subjects involved in the study from which data is entered and results are calculated. The larger the n is in a study, the more likely that the study will have reliable and repeatable results.

TABLE 7

TOXICITY GRADING OF DOGS AND CATS RECEIVING CHEMOTHERAPY

Toxic Effect and Grade	Signs
Anorexia	
1 (mild)	< 2 day's duration
2 (moderate)	≥ 2 but < 5 day's duration
3 (severe)	≥ 5 day's duration, 10%weight loss
Vomiting	
1 (mild)	1 to 5 episodes per day; < 2 days
2 (moderate)	6 to 10 episodes per day
3 (severe)	Intractable; requires hospitalization
Diarrhea	
1 (mild)	3 to 7 watery stools per day; < 2 days
2 (moderate)	> 7 watery stools per day
3 (severe)	> Bloody stools; requires hospitalization
Neutropenia	
1 (mild)	Segmented neutrophils > 2,000 and < 3,000/μL
2 (moderate)	Segmented neutrophils > 1,000 and < 2,000/μL
3 (severe)	Segmented neutrophils < 1,000/μL
Thrombocytopenia	
1 (mild)	Platelets > 100,000 and < 200,000/μL
2 (moderate)	Platelets > 30,000 and < 100,000/μL
3 (severe)	Platelets < 30,000/μL

From Moore AS, Cotter SM, Frimbgerger AE, Wood CA, Rand WM, L'Hureux DA. A comparison of doxorubicin and COP for maintenance of remission in cats with lymphoma. J Vet Intern Med 1996;10:372-375.

PRETREATMENT PROGNOSTIC FACTORS

Dogs

Prognostic factors are variables that independently influence the response and the duration of that response to a particular treatment. Some of the variables evaluated in veterinary medicine for prognostic significance include sex, neuter status, age, body weight, breed, World Health Organization (WHO) stage, WHO substage, prior administration of corticosteroids, paraneoplastic conditions, initial response to chemotherapy, chromosomal abnormalities, histologic classification and and immunophenotype. Unfortunately, few of the physical or clinical factors evaluated have consistently been associated with a given prognosis. However, commonly agreed on prognostic factors that negatively affect remission and survival in dogs with lymphoma include substage B, the presence of hypercalcemia, mediastinal lymph node involvement, T cell phenotype, and cutaneous, central nervous system, or renal involvement.[2,20,2,26,37-39,65,84-93]

Cats

Generally agreed on prognostic factors that negatively affect remission and survival in cats with lymphoma include substage B, positive FeLV and/or FIV test status, spinal, cutaneous or renal involvement, hypercalcemia, and T cell phenotype.[1,94] Cats seem to be especially susceptible to anorexia with gastrointestinal lymphoma and following chemotherapy with doxorubicin so a willingness by the owner and attending clinician to provide enteral or parenteral nutrition can be critical to treatment outcome.

Chemotherapy Options for Treatment

SINGLE DRUG PROTOCOLS

Single drug protocols are rarely used except in instances where the financial demands of a more aggressive protocol cannot be overcome or when a more aggressive combination chemotherapy protocol will put the patient at risk for a serious cytopenia and/or sepsis.

Dogs

Prednisone alone has been reported to provide a complete remission or partial remission in about 50% of the dogs with a mean remission/survival time of 30-60 days. This essentially is no increase in survival compared to untreated dogs. While response is not long, it is successful, and the dogs "feel better".[41,95] However, an advantage of single agent prednisone as treatment of lymphoma is that no monitoring of peripheral blood cell counts is necessary, and the patients are likely to die from lymphoma long before the side effects of chronic glucocorticoid administration becomes an issue.

The wisdom of using prednisone alone has been questioned, because it may blunt the response and remission length if more aggressive chemotherapy drugs are used later. A provocative report in 1991 found 39% of dogs (11/28) treated with glucocorticoids before starting a combination chemotherapy protocol had shorter remissions than those dogs not given glucocorticoids (134 days versus 267 days, respectively).[96]

Doxorubicin is the most effective drug that can be used alone to treat lymphoma in dogs (Table 8). The complete response rate for dogs with lymphoma treated with doxorubicin alone ranges from 41% to 76%, and the median duration of first remission ranges from 52-219 days (mean of 190 days).[96-101] The median survival time using doxorubicin as single agent therapy has been reported as 100-300 days, and the mean survival time using doxorubicin as single agent therapy is reported to range from 265-362 days.[96-101] In one study of 58 dogs with lymphoma treated with doxorubicin alone, 17% of the dogs that achieved a complete remission were still in the first remission at 1 year. In the same study, 33% of all dogs treated were alive at 1 year, and 10% were alive at 2 years.[98]

TABLE 8	
SINGLE AGENT DOXORUBICIN FOR DOGS WITH LYMPHOMA	
Drug and Dose	**Schedule**
Doxorubicin 30 mg/m² IV for dogs weighing over 10 kg. 1 mg/kg for dogs weighing under 10 kg	Given as bolus with 5% dextrose and water drip on day 1 every 3 weeks for 4-6 treatments. **Always** use a patent catheter for administration

Comment
A cardiac evaluation including echocardiogram is advised prior to initial treatment and when close to 180mg/m² total cumulative dose
Pre-treat with diphenhydramine

Epirubicin is an analog of doxorubicin. It differs from doxorubicin only by changing the hydroxyl group on C4 of the sugar moiety from an axial to an equitorial position.[102] This is enough of a molecular change to decrease the cardiotoxicity in both humans and dogs.[103,104] In a clinical trial of dogs with lymphoma at Purdue University that were given 6 or more treatments of doxorubicin or epirubicin, significantly less cardiotoxicity was seen, both clinically and histologically, in dogs treated with epirubicin.[98,105] Dogs treated with both drugs in comparative studies had a similar response to therapy, duration of remission, and survival times.[98,100,105,106] Epirubicin is currently available in the United States as the drug Ellence, and in Europe as the drug Pharmorubicin®, but it is very expensive.

Mitoxantrone as single agent therapy for previously treated and previously untreated dogs with lymphoma is not as effective as doxorubicin. The complete remission rate for 74 dogs treated with mitoxantrone was only 26%. Of the 40 dogs in this study that were previously untreated, only 10 achieved complete remission with median duration of remission of 94 days. For the 34 dogs previously treated with other drugs, only 9 achieved a complete remission with median duration of remission of 126 days.[107] Mitoxantrone, though not as effective, can be used as a substitute for doxorubicin for dogs with or predisposed to cardiac disease.

Cats

Less is published on single drug protocols for cats, but extrapolations from experience can be made. Prednisone alone will often induce partial or complete remissions in cats with mediastinal or multicentric lymphoma. Prednisone alone is less successful when treating alimentary and cutaneous involvent. However, in circumstances when owners are unable or unwilling to provide more appropriate combination chemotherapy, prednisone can be of great value to the well being of the patient even if only for a short time.

Doxorubicin as a lone agent for lymphoma in cats has been reported sparingly. Two separate reports suggest very ineffective and inconsistent responses to doxorubicin when used alone. In one study of 19 cases, 5 cats achieved a complete response to doxorubicin with a median duration of remission of 92 days (range, 54-575 days). As expected, cats testing FeLV negative had longer survival than FeLV test positive cats. Loss of appetite was a common toxicity and was observed in 9/19 cats in this series.[107a, 107b]

Doxorubicin has been shown to be more effective when given as a single agent to maintain remission of cats already in a complete remission with COP chemotherapy. Cats receiving doxorubicin for maintenance chemotherapy had median duration of remission of 281 days (n=7) vs. a median duration of remission of 83 days (n=11) for cats receiving the combination protocol as maintenance chemotherapy.[83]

Idarubicin is an anthracycline derivative (similar to doxorubicin and epirubicin) that is available for use by parenteral and oral routes. Oral administration of an effective chemotherapy protocol in cats can be attractive in some patients. Most cats tolerate a dose of 2 mg/day for three consecutive days every 21 days.[108] One published study of idarubicin in 18 cats with lymphoma after complete remission was established with a combination protocol found that the median duration of remission was 183 days which compares favorably with other protocols.[109]

Methorexate is a part of several published protocols for cats with lymphoma. However, it may be ineffective in cats with lymphoma.[108,110,111]

The use of anabolic steroids in cats has been popular from time to time as a presumed stimulant to general well being and to appetite. There is no evidence to suggest that anabolic steroids for these uses are of benefit.

COMBINATION CHEMOTHERAPY

While single drugs are effective, most protocols employ a multiple drug approach. The theory behind multi-drug protocols is that the simultaneous use of drugs with different mechanism of actions which are effective at different parts of the cell cycle will achieve a more efficient cell kill and develop less drug resistance. Drugs used in multi-drug protocols must be effective as single agents against a given tumor type, they must be used in compatible and correct schedules, they should have different mechanisms of action, and they should not have overlapping toxicities. The majority of multi-drug protocols have induction and maintenance phases. Induction drugs are used in the beginning of the protocol and usually have a rapid effect on tumor cell populations. The maintenance drugs tend to be orally administered, used alone or with intermittent injections of intravenous drugs, continued for months to years once remission is obtained. A number of useful combination chemotherapy protocols for aggressive, high-grade lymphoma are given in Tables 9 to 15.

Dogs

Many of the combination protocols used in dogs are based on the combination of cyclophosphamide, vincristine and prednisone, with or without doxorubicin. The combination protocols with the longest duration of remission included doxorubicin.[1]

There are many protocols know by the acronym COP (Cytoxan® {cyclophosphamide}, Oncovin® {vincristine}, prednisone). One version of COP consists of cyclophosphamide, vincristine and prednisone is given for 6 weeks of induction followed by a maintenance protocol of methotrexate, higher dose cyclophosphamide and lower dose prednisone for an additional 6 weeks.[97] The cycle continues for 1 year using 6 weeks of maintenance followed by 1 week of induction, in a repeating cycle (Table 9). The reported median first remission for 67 dogs on the above COP protocol was only 45 days, but remission was measured from the time of first response (up to several weeks post initiation of chemotherapy) to relapse. Complete remissions (35/67) and partial remissions (11/67) were achieved in 69% of the dogs. Median survival time was 123 days and was measured from the time of first chemotherapy until death.[97] The many versions of COP in use in veterinary oncology all seem to produce similar results.

Cotter et al reported on a COP-based protocol alone as induction then adding doxorubicin to the 3 drugs as the maintenance phase (COPA).[39] These dogs were compared to historical controls that had been treated with a version of COP. Complete remission occurred in 75% (58/77) of the COP and 83% (38/46) of the dogs treated with COPA. The median duration of remission was 6 months for COP treated dogs and 7 months for the COPA-treated dogs. Median survival times were not reported, but 19% (11/77) of the COP-treated dogs and 26% (10/46) of the COPA-treated dogs were alive at 1 year.

TABLE 9
COP FOR DOGS WITH LYMPHOMA

INDUCTION Therapy is given weekly for 6 consecutive weeks

Drugs and Dosages	Schedule
Vincristine 0.5-0.7 mg/m^2 IV	Day 1 of each week
Cyclophosphamide 50 mg/m^2 PO SID	Day 4, 5, 6, and 7 of each week
Prednisone 20 mg/m^2 PO BID	For all 6 weeks

Comments

Monitor CBC, platelet count and measure lymph nodes on 1st day of therapy.

Note that you should not break a cyclophosphamide tablet. If significant toxicity occurs, give dose every 2-3 days, or if hemorrhagic cystitis occurs, chlorambucil may be substituted: 50 mg of cyclophosphamide = 8 mg of chlorambucil.

MAINTENANCE Therapy is given weekly for 6 consecutive weeks

Drugs and Dosages	Schedule
Methotrexate 5.0 mg/m^2 PO SID	Days 1 and 5 of each week
Cyclophosphamide 100 mg/m^2 PO SID	Day 3 of each week
Prednisone 20 mg/m^2 PO QOD	For all 6 weeks

Comments

If the dog is in complete remission after first 6 weeks of maintenance therapy, repeat induction therapy for 1 week.

Follow 1 week of induction with 6 weeks of maintenance, then repeat with 1 week induction, etc.

This regimen is followed for at least 1 year if complete remission is maintained

Re-evaluate the dog each 7th week to try and identify early relapse.

If relapse is observed several weeks to months after induction, the same protocol can be used to try reinduction.

If vomiting or anorexia occurs with methotrexate, check the dose. If the dose/tablet is too high, consider having the drug compounded into a capsule with the exact dose needed. If the dose is correct but the dog will not tolerate the drug, cytosine arabinoside may be substituted: 5 mg methotrexate = 100 mg cytosine arabinoside.

It is not usually necessary to monitor cell counts weekly.

Strive to maintain blood cell counts as follows:

WBC > 4.0 x 10^3 PMN > 3.0 x 10^3 Platelet > 100.0 x 10^3

One published protocol that was evaluated in 147 dogs with lymphoma was basically a combination chemotherapy protocol that alternates different single agents weekly (vincristine, cyclophosphamide, methotrexate).[111] The exception was when vincristine and L-asparaginase were both given in the first week. A complete response was seen in 77% of the dogs, and a partial response was seen in 18%. Median duration of remission for dogs in complete remission was 140 days. Median survival for all responding dogs was 265 days. Median survival for dogs with complete remission was 290 days, while median survival for dogs with partial remission was 152 days.[111]

Some protocols have better published survival data but it is important to carefully evaluate the studies for toxicity, mortality, dose reductions, and/or early termination of the protocols. For example, a protocol designated as ACOPA was evaluated in 41 dogs with lymphoma.[112] This protocol is similar to the COPA protocol, but L-asparaginase is given with vincristine for the first 4 weeks of induction. A complete remission was seen in 76% of the dogs, and a partial remission occurred in 12 % of dogs. Duration of remission for dogs in complete remission was 334 days. Median survival for the dogs in complete remission was 365 days. Median survival for dogs in partial remission was 91 days. Thirteen dogs (48%) were alive and in remission at 1 year.[112] However attractive ACOPA may at first seem in terms of remission and survival, it is also fairly toxic to patients because of the drug doses employed and is not recommended.

In the COPA and the ACOPA protocols, cyclophosphamide and vincristine are given at very high doses (250-300 mg/m^2 and 0.75 mg/m^2, respectively). Toxicity was greater for the ACOPA protocol with 15/41 (37%) of the dogs having vomiting, diarrhea, anorexia, lethargy or pyrexia. Twelve of the 41 (29%) dogs required hospitalization during the first 4 weeks of therapy. During induction, 4 dogs died acutely. Less toxicity was reported with therapy after induction was completed. Doses of cyclophosphamide above 200 mg/m^2 and 0.7 mg/m^2 of vincristine will routinely produce unnecessary toxicity and should not be administered. Because of unwarranted toxicity, protocols containing these drugs at these high doses cannot be recommended.

A more useful protocol for canine lymphoma is known as COPLA (Table 10). This protocol uses the same drugs as the more aggressive protocols but in a different sequence and with slightly lower

TABLE 10

COPLA FOR DOGS WITH LYMPHOMA[112A]

INDUCTION

Drugs and Dosages	Schedule
L-asparaginase 10,000 IU/ m² SQ	Day 1 of weeks 1 and 2

Comments

Monitor CBC, platelet count and measure lymph nodes on first day of therapy

Pre-treat with diphenhydramine prior to therapy

Drugs and Dosages	Schedule
Vincristine 0.5-0.7 mg/m² IV	Day 1 of each week for 8 consecutive weeks
Cyclophosphamide 50 mg/m² PO QOD	For 8 weeks
Prednisone 20 mg/m² PO SID	For 1st week, then QOD for 2-5 weeks, then drop dose to 10 mg/m² PO QOD for weeks 6-12
Doxorubicin 30 mg/m² IV for dogs weighing over 10 kg. 1 mg/kg for dogs weighing under 10 kg	Given day 1 on weeks 6, 9, 12

Comments

A cardiac evaluation including echocardiogram is advised prior to initial treatment and when close to 180mg/m² total cumulative dose

Pre-treat with diphenhydramine

MAINTENANCE

Drugs and Dosages	Schedule
Vincristine 0.5-0.7 mg/m² IV	Day 1 every other week for 2 times, then day 1 every 3rd week for 3 times, then day 1 every 4th week for 4 times, then day 1 every 6th week for 1 year
Chlorambucil 4 mg/m² PO QOD	Start on week 9 and continue for up to 2 years if complete remission is maintained

Comments

Try to maintain cell counts as follows:

WBC > 4.0 x10³   PMN > 3.0 x10³   Platelet >100.0 x10³

dosages. Remission and survival times are in the range of most combination protocols (180 and 270 days respectively), but the number of dogs achieving a complete or partial remission is high. It is an extremely well tolerated protocol but like most combination protocols requires frequent office visits and laboratory monitoring.[112a]

A very popular treatment protocol that was developed at the University of Wisconsin-Madison (UW-M) reports to have some of the longest remission and survival times for dogs with lymphoma with what many clinicians find as acceptable toxicity (Table 11). Keller, et al, reported on 55 dogs with lymphoma treated with a

TABLE 11
ORIGINAL UNIVERSITY WISCONSIN-MADISON PROTOCOL**

INDUCTION Week One

Drugs and Dosages	Schedule
L-asparaginase 400 IU/ kg IM	Day 1 of week 1
Vincristine 0.7 mg/m² IV	Day 1 week 1
Prednisone 2 mg/kg PO SID	Daily

Comments

Monitor CBC, platelet count and measure lymph nodes on first day of therapy. Try to maintain cell counts during chemotherapy as follows: WBC > 4.0 x10³   PMN > 3.0 x10³   Platelet >100.0 x10³

INDUCTION Week Two

Cyclophosphamide 200 mg/m² IV	Day 1 of week 2
Prednisone 1.5 mg/kg PO SID	Daily

Comments

Do not exceed maximum dose of 250 mg of cyclophosphamide. Consider giving furosemide to reduce the potential for urothelial toxicity

INDUCTION Week Three

Vincristine 0.7 mg/m² IV

Prednisone 1 mg/kg PO SID

INDUCTION Week Four

Doxorubicin 30 mg/m² IV for dogs weighing over 10 kg. 1 mg/kg for dogs weighing under 10 kg

Comments

A cardiac evaluation including echocardiogram is advised prior to initial treatment and when close to 180mg/m² total cumulative dose. Pre-treat with diphenhydramine

TABLE 11

CONTINUED

INDUCTION Week Five

Drugs and Dosages

No Treatment

INDUCTION Week Six

Vincristine 0.7 mg/m² IV

INDUCTION Week Seven

Cyclophosphamide 200 mg/m² IV

Comments

Do not exceed maximum dose of 250 mg of cyclophosphamide.

Consider giving furosemide to reduce the potential for urothelial toxicity

INDUCTION Week Eight

Vincristine 0.7 mg/m² IV

INDUCTION Week Nine

Doxorubicin 30 mg/m² IV for dogs weighing over 10 kg. 1 mg/kg for dogs weighing under 10 kg

INDUCTION Week Ten

No Treatment

MAINTENANCE Week Eleven - One Hundred Four

Vincristine 0.7 mg/m² IV

Chlorambucil 1.4 mg/kg PO

Methotrexate 0.8 mg/kg IV

or

Doxorubicin 30 mg/m² IV for dogs weighing over 10 kg. 1 mg/kg for dogs weighing under 10 kg

Comments

Alternate these three treatments every two weeks. After week 25 alternate these three treatments every 3 weeks. After week 49 alternate these three treatments every 4 weeks. All drugs are discontinued after 2 years if the dog remains in complete remission.

A cardiac evaluation including echocardiogram is advised prior to initial treatment and when close to 180mg/m² total cumulative dose. Pre-treat with diphenhydramine

Do not exceed a total cumulative dose of 180-200 mg/m² doxorubicin

**From: Vail DM. Treatment and prognosis of canine malignant lymphoma. In: Bonagura JD, Kirk RW. Kirk's current veterinary therapy XII small animal practice. Philadelphia. W B Saunders Co. 1995;494-497
Overall response rate = 91% (CR plus PR)
Median duration of remission = 36 weeks
Median survival = 51 weeks

sequential drug protocol of vincristine, L-asparaginase, chlorambucil, methotrexate, and doxorubicin.[113] Treatment is continued for 3 years or until relapse. The overall response rate for this protocol was 91% with 84% of dogs achieving a complete remission and 7% of dogs achieving a partial remission. The median duration of remission for all dogs responding was 252 days and the median survival was 357 days. In contrast to the ACOPA protocol (that is composed of the same drugs, but at different doses and schedule) no life threatening toxicity was reported with induction, and no dogs died of treatment related causes. However, drug dosages were adjusted in 40% of the dogs due to gastrointestinal upset or neutropenia. Of the dogs that had achieved a complete or partial remission, 43% were still in remission at 1 year, and 25% were in remission at 2 years.[113] Over time, the Wisconsin protocol has evolved in response to reported side effects and the current version of the protocol is given in Table 12. Note that adjustments in dose are made by the primary clinician based on patient tolerance of the aggressive drug doses.

A similar protocol used in two studies that combined either native aspiraginase or asparaginase conjugated to polyethylene glycol (PEG asparaginase) with vincristine, cyclophosphamide, doxorubicin, methotrexate, and decreasing doses of prednisone, also produced high response rates, remission duration, and survival.[114] During the first 2 weeks, the L-asparaginase was used alone, then the other drugs were added. Complete remission rates for 69 dogs were reported as 86-94% (30/35 dogs and 32/34 dogs, respectively), with median disease-free intervals of 214-217 days. The median survival times were 319-356 days. In these studies, 10% were long-term survivors and considered cured.[113,114] Actual cures following chemotherapy are very rare and a 10% reported cure rate in a small population of patients without lifelong follow-up is suspect.

A reliable protocol that still enjoys popularity because of its efficacy and safety was developed at the Animal Medical Center in New York City in the 1980s (Table 13). The overall median survival for dogs treated with this protocol is reported to be 10 months, with survival in excess of 12 months in 30% of patients.[115]

TABLE 12

UPDATED UNIVERSITY WISCONSIN-MADISON PROTOCOL**

INDUCTION Week One

Drugs and Dosages	Schedule
L-asparaginase 400 IU/ kg IM	Day 1 of week 1
Vincristine 0.5-.7 mg/m² IV use lower dose down if side effects unacceptable at higher dose	Day 1 of week 1

Comments

Monitor CBC, platelet count and measure lymph nodes on first day of therapy. Try to maintain cell counts during chemotherapy as follows: WBC > 4.0 x10³   PMN > 3.0 x10³   Platelet >100.0 x10³

INDUCTION Week Two

Prednisone 1.5 mg/kg PO SID	Daily for 7 days
Cyclophosphamide 250 mg/m² IV	Day 1 of week 2

Comments

Consider giving with furoesmide to reduce potential for urothelial toxicity

INDUCTION Week Three

Prednisone 1.0mg/kg PO SID	
Vincristine 0.5-0.7 mg/m² IV use lower dose down if side effects unacceptable at higher dose	

INDUCTION Week Four

Doxorubicin 30 mg/m² IV for dogs weighing over 10 kg. 1 mg/kg for dogs weighing under 10 kg	
Prednisone 0.5 mg/kg PO SID	

Comments

A cardiac evaluation including echocardiogram is advised prior to initial treatment and when close to 180mg/m² total cumulative dose. Pre-treat with diphenhydramine

INDUCTION Week Five

No Treatment	

INDUCTION Week Six

Vincristine 0.5-0.7 mg/m² IV use lower dose down if side effects unacceptable at higher dose	

INDUCTION Week Seven

Cyclophosphamide 250 mg/m² IV	Day 1 of week 7

continued

TABLE 12	
CONTINUED	

Comments	
Consider giving with furoesmide to reduce potential for urothelial toxicity	
INDUCTION Week Eight	
Vincristine 0.5-0.7 mg/m² IV use lower dose down if side effects unacceptable at higher dose	
INDUCTION Week Nine	
Doxorubicin 30 mg/m² IV for dogs weighing over 10 kg. 1 mg/kg for dogs weighing under 10 kg	
Cyclophosphamide 200 mg/m² IV	
Comments	
Consider giving with furoesmide to reduce potential for urothelial toxicity	
Vincristine 0.7 mg/m² IV	
Doxorubicin 30 mg/m² IV for dogs weighing over 10 kg. 1 mg/kg for dogs weighing under 10 kg	
Comments	
A cardiac evaluation including echocardiogram is advised prior to initial treatment and when close to 180mg/m² total cumulative dose. Pre-treat with diphenhydramine	
INDUCTION Week Ten	
No Treatment	
MAINTENANCE Week Eleven - Twenty	
Repeat of weeks 6-9	
Comments	
If in complete remission, stop treatment until relapse (usually between 2 and 9 months). Once relapse is documented, begin again.	

*** Helfand S. Personal communication, 2003.

TABLE 13	
OLD ANIMAL MEDICAL CENTER PROTOCOL*	

INDUCTION Week One

Drugs and Dosages	Schedule
L-asparaginase 10,000 IU/m² IM	Day 1 of week 1
Vincristine 0.7 mg/m² IV	Day 1 of week 1
Prednisone 30 mg/m² PO SID	Daily

TABLE 13

CONTINUED

INDUCTION Week One

Drugs and Dosages

Comments

Monitor CBC, platelet count and measure lymph nodes on first day of therapy. Try to maintain cell counts during chemotherapy as follows: WBC > 4.0 x10^3 PMN > 3.0 x10^3 Platelet >100.0 x10^3

INDUCTION Week Two

Cyclophosphamide 200 mg/m^2 IV	Day 1 of week 2

Comments

Maximum dose of 250 mg cyclophosphamide. Consider giving furoesmide to reduce the potential for urothelial toxicity

Prednisone 20 mg/m^2 PO SID	Daily

INDUCTION Week Three

Doxorubicin 30 mg/m^2 IV for dogs weighing over 10 kg. 1 mg/kg for dogs weighing under 10 kg	

Comments

A cardiac evaluation including echocardiogram is advised prior to initial treatment and when close to 180mg/m^2 total cumulative dose. Pre-treat with diphenhydramine

Prednisone 10 mg/m^2 PO SID	

INDUCTION Week Four - Six

Same as weeks 1-3 except discontinue asparaginase and prednisone	

MAINTENANCE Week Eight

Vincristine 0.7 mg/m^2 IV	
Cyclophosphamide 200 mg/m^2 IV Maximum dose of 250 mg	
Vincristine 0.7 mg/m^2 IV	
Methotrexate 0.5 mg/kg IV Maximum dose of 25 mg	

Repeat weeks 8-14 for one year if complete remission is maintained. After one year repeat this sequence every three weeks for 6 months, then once a month for an additional 6 months if complete remission is maintained. Consider giving furoesmide to reduce the potential for urothelial toxicity

*Reported overall median survival = 10 months for dogs and 7 months for cats. Survival > 12 months in 30% of patients

Modified from: Matus RE. Chemotherapy of lymphoma and leukemia. In: Kirk RW, ed. Current Veterinary Therapy X. Philadelphia. WB Saunders 1989;482-488.

For a histologically low-grade lymphoma, a milder form of chemotherapy should be employed. Because these types of lymphoma tend not to respond to aggressive chemotherapy protocols, they are not likely to achieve a long-term remission. The goal for treatment of low-grade lymphoma is to make the dogs feel better and stay as "happy and healthy" for as long as possible. This is best achieved with drugs like chlorambucil (Leukeran®) (4 mg/m^2 every 48 hours) and prednisone (20 mg/m^2 every 48 hours) or a COP protocol (see Table 9). Usually some reduction of lymph node size or decrease in severity of clinical signs is seen, but the most important clinical change is often in the dog's attitude.

Similarly, a less aggressive start to a protocol is advocated by some oncologists for sick dogs with severe gastrointestinal or bone marrow involvement. A 'gentle' initial week or two of therapy (vincristine, prednisone, ± L-asparaginase) may decrease the tumor burden enough to allow the dog to 'feel better' and be able to tolerate any side effects from a more aggressive protocol. The author rarely uses this approach unless the patient is extremely debilitated.

The choice of a protocol depends on the needs of the owner and patient and unfortunately, sometimes, on financial and time constraints. For owners that decline to use a complex and aggressive protocol, single agent doxorubicin can be effective, easy to administer, requires only a visit to the office every 3 weeks, is relatively inexpensive, and has no overlapping toxicities to worry about (see Table 8). Remission and survival times are good when up to 4-6 treatments are given and allow the owner and pet some good quality time at home. Approximately 33% of the dogs are alive at one year with this treatment.[94] Alternatively, a COP protocol can be equally effective and it is often virtually free of side effects an owner could detect when used at recommended doses (see Table 9).

Cats

Most of the combination protocols used to treat feline lymphoma are based on cyclophosphamide, vincristine and prednisone (COP).[1,94,116,1184] A number of variations on the COP theme have been published, with success of the protocol depending as much on the anatomic form treated and the FeLV test status as on the protocol itself.[109,115-119] Most of the multi-drug chemotherapy protocols induced complete remission in 60-70% of cats with all forms of lymphoma.[57,58,94,116,118] Reported median remission times for combination protocols range from 83-281days.[114,116, 118] Median survival times for combination protocols range from 49-209 days with approximately 30% alive at 1 year.[56,58,90,116,118]

One early study in a small number of cats reported mediastinal lymphoma (n=12) and multicentric (n= 4) as being very responsive to treatment (92% and 100%, respectively) and having median remission times of 6 months and 5 months, respectively. The protocol consisted of vincristine and cyclophosphamide given every 3 weeks and prednisone given daily with the whole protocol continuing for 1 year.[116]

In separate studies, 28 cats with alimentary lymphoma and 9 cats with spinal lymphoma did not respond as well to COP therapy. Only 33 % of the cats with alimentary lymphoma and 50% of the cats with spinal lymphoma achieved a complete remission.[68,115] Median remission time for cats with spinal lymphoma was 98 days.[115] Cats with alimentary lymphoma that achieved a complete remission had a median duration of remission of 213 days. However, the median survival for all cats with alimentary lymphoma was only 50 days.[115]

A different study of 21 FeLV test negative cats with alimentary lymphoma treated with a combination of prednisone, L-asparaginase, vincristine, cyclophosphamide, doxorubicin, and methotrexate reported a median survival of 40 weeks (range, 4 to 120 weeks).[116] Interestingly, cats that achieved complete remission did not have significantly longer median survival time than did cats that only achieved a partial response. Immunophenotyping was performed on 13 of the tumors in this study; 10 were T-cell type and 3 were B-cell type. There was no difference in survival or response to chemotherapy between cats with T-cell or B-cell types of lymphoma in this study. The results of this study suggest that most cats with alimentary lymphoma that are FeLV test negative will respond better to chemotherapy than was reported in earlier studies.[116]

In a report of 75 cats with various forms of lymphoma treated with a protocol consisting of vincristine, cyclophosphamide, methotrexate, and vincristine was given at weeks 1 and 3, cyclophosphamide at week 2, methotrexate at week 4, and prednisone was used if there was mediastinal involvement or the cat was not responding or had relapsed.[117] Treatment was continued for 2 years or until relapse. Sixteen of the 75 cats in this study with multicentric lymphoma had a response rate of 68% and the median remission length of 18 months.[117]

In a similar protocol that added L-asparaginase at week 1 of induction in 103 cats with lymphoma, median survival was 210 days with a 62% (64/103) complete remission rate, where complete remission was defined as ≥ 75% reduction in volume of tumor.[94] Cats with an FeLV positive test had shorter survival times but still responded to therapy well. Of the cats that achieved a complete response as defined in this study, 30% were alive at 1 year.[94]

In a different study of 28 cats with renal lymphoma treated with a similar protocol, 17 cats (61%) achieved a complete remission with median remission length of 127 days.[57] Ten of the 28 cats with renal lymphoma had cytosine arabinoside added to their maintenance protocol and none developed CNS relapse, while 40% of the remaining cats not treated with cytosine arabinoside developed CNS lymphoma.[55]

The most recent large study of cats with lymphoma treated with COP was conducted in the Netherlands, a country with a low prevalence of FeLV. In this study, 22 cats had mediastinal lymphoma, 11 had alimentarly localization, 7 had multicentric disease, 8 had nasal lymphoma, and 13 had extranodal (miscellaneous) lymphoma. Complete remission was acheived in 46 of 61 cats, and the estimated 1 and 2 year disease free periods of the 46 cats in CR was 51.4% and 37.8% respectively. The median survival time and 1 year survival rate for cats with mediastinal lymphoma were 262 days and 49.9% respectively.[4]

The author recommends a standard COP protocol described in Table 14 for cats with most forms of lymphoma. Cats tolerate the drugs and doses in this protocol very well. Side effects with this version of COP are negligible, and the remission times are good. Side effects, if seen at all, usually occur during the induction phase. Since most drugs in this COP protocol are given orally, dosage or schedule adjustments are easily made. Supportive care is not usually needed. While the author has not personally used doxorubicin as maintenance for lymphoma, one report of COP followed by doxorubicin (Table 15) showed dramatically better remission times and bears consideration.[83] Use this protocol cautiously because of the high doses required of vincristine (0.75 mg/m^2 IV) and cyclophosphamide (300mg/m^2 IV). If the total tumor burden is large and needs to be decreased in size quickly, L-asparaginase may be added into the COP protocol at the beginning of the therapy (day 1) for 1-2 treatments.

TABLE 14
COP FOR CATS WITH LYMPHOMA

INDUCTION Therapy is given weekly for 6 consecutive weeks

Drugs and Dosages	Schedule
Vincristine 0.5-0.7 mg/m^2 IV	Day 1 of each week
Comments	
Monitor CBC, platelet count and measure lymph nodes on first day of therapy	
Cyclophosphamide 50 mg/m^2 PO SID	Day 4, 5, 6, & 7 of each week
Comments	
Do not break tablet	
Prednisone 20 mg/m^2 PO BID	For all 6 weeks

MAINTENANCE Therapy is given weekly for 6 consecutive weeks

Methotrexate 5.0 mg/m^2 PO SID	Days 1 and 5 of each week

Comments

If vomiting or anorexia occurs with methotrexate, check the dose to make sure cat is not being overdosed. If the dose/tablet is too high, consult pharmacist and have tablet recompounded into capsule for proper dose. If dose is correct but cat intolerant of drug, cytosine arabinoside may be substituted: 5 mg methotrexate = 100 mg cytosine arabinoside

Not usually necessary to monitor cell counts weekly

Desired cell counts:

WBC > 4.0 x 10^3 PMN > 3.0 x 10^3 Platelet >100.0 x 10^3

Cyclophosphamide 100 mg/m^2 PO SID	Day 3 of each week
Prednisone 20 mg/m^2 PO QOD	For all 6 weeks

TABLE 15

COP AND DOX FOR CATS WITH LYMPHOMA

INDUCTION COP Induction protocol is repeated weekly for 4 consecutive weeks. Then maintenance with doxorubicin is started.

Drugs and Dosages	Schedule
Vincristine 0.75 mg/m² IV through a patent catheter	Day 1 of each week
Comments	
Monitor CBC, platelet count and measure lymph nodes on first day of therapy	
Cyclophosphamide 300 mg/m² IV through a patent catheter	Given every 3 weeks, same day as vincristine
Prednisone 40 mg/m² PO SID	For all 4 weeks
Comments	
Consider giving furoesmide to reduce the potential for urothelial toxicity. Use this protocol with caution due to high suggested doses of vincristine and cyclophohamide.	

MAINTENANCE DOX Doxorubicin is given every 3 weeks for 5 months (7 total treatments) or until relapse

Doxorubicin 25 mg/m² IV through a patent catheter	Given every 3 weeks
Comments	
Cardiac evaluation (including echocardiogram) is recommended prior to each treatment and before last if close to 150 mg/m² total cumulative dose. Monitor CBC and platelet count	
Monthly serum biochemistry panel	
ECG prior to each treatment with doxorubicin	
Echocardiogram before first and after last treatment with doxorubicin	

Potential Complications of Chemotherapy

CUTANEOUS TOXICITY

The skin is occasionally affected by chemotherapy. One of the most damaging cutaneous reactions to chemotherapy occurs when a caustic drug that is intended for intravenous administration is given in, or leaks into, the perivascular tissue. Drugs that can cause severe cutaneous reactions include doxorubicin, vincristine, and vinblastine.[120] These drugs cause acute local tissue necrosis that is very difficult to treat once it has happened (Figure 14). The best treatment is avoidance by the religious use of carefully placed and patent intravenous catheter used each and every time an intravenous chemotherapy is given.

Mild to moderate hypersensitivity reactions occur approximately 10% of the time during the administration of doxorubicin (Figures 15 and 16). The angioedema, uticaria, and pruritis that characterize this

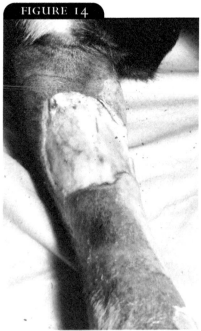

FIGURE 14

Figure 14. Acute Tissue Necrosis and Skin Sloughing Secondary to Extravasation of Doxorubicin into Perivascular Tissue. This complication is avoidable with the use of a carefully placed intravenous vascular catheter for the administration of cytotoxic drugs.

Figure 15. Acute Hypersensitivity Reaction that Occurred During the Administration of Doxorubicin to a Dog. Note the small raised areas of edema in the skin (wheel formation). Doxorubicin may cause rapid degranulation of mast cells within the skin and cause cutaneous hypersensitivity reactions.

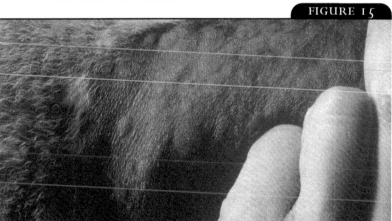

FIGURE 15

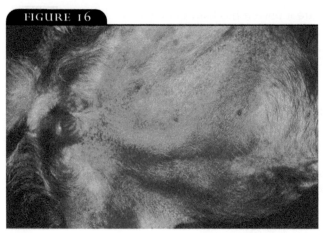

FIGURE 16

The red skin on the abdomen of this dog represents another manifestation of an acute hypersensitivity reaction occurring during administration of doxorubicin.

reaction are attributed to histamine release from degranulating mast cells in the skin in response to doxorubicin exposure. A rapid rise in plasma histamine concentration following doxorubicin administration has been documented in dogs.[120-122]

Cutaneous reactions to doxorubicin can be mitigated in most cases by pretreatment with corticosteroids (1mg/kg dexamethasone sodium phosphate and 2-4 mg/kg diphenhydramine, IV prior to doxorubicin use).

Alopecia is another, but uncommon, side effect of doxorubicin use in dogs. One study found that 2 of 85 dogs developed alopecia following doxorubicin administration (Figure 17).[123] Melanosis of the skin (increased pigmentation) is also infrequently observed in dogs treated with doxorubicin.[123] Although rare, increased melanin pigmentation most often occurs in the axilla and inguinal regions.

MYELOSUPPRESSION

Almost all drugs used in cancer chemotherapy result in some degree of myelosuppression. Notable exceptions include L-asparaginase and corticosteroids. Myelosuppression is usually characterized by a rapid decrease in circulating neutrophils and platelets that will normally return to reference ranges prior to the next sched-

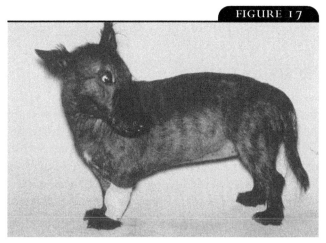

FIGURE 17

Alopecia primarily on the trunk of a dog treated with doxorubicin. Breeds of dogs with hair growth cycle in constant anagen phase such as poodles are more susceptible to alopecia than dogs that have the more usual hair growth cycle of a prolonged telogen phase in addition to a relatively short anagen phase of hair growth.

uled cycle of drug(s) in most protocols. The degree, duration, and consequences of the myelosuppression varies with the individual drug, dose, residual normal bone marrow stem cell population, and general health of the patient.

The most relevant manifestations of myelosupprssion following chemotherapy are neurtopenia and thrombocytopenia. Life-threatening sepsis and/or bleeding are possible with severe neutropenia and/or thrombocytopenia. The nadir for neutorphil numbers in dogs and cats treated with common drugs used for chemotherapy is usually between 7 and 10 days. The nadir for platelet numbers in dogs and cats treated with chemotherapy is usually a few days earlier than the neutrophil nadir.[124,125] Myelosuppression can be graded according to Table 7. Changes in dose or dosing interval may be required if toxicity is unacceptable.

ANEMIA

Anemia is rarely a clinically significant side effect of chemotherapy. However, a mild progressive anemia is a common finding for patients receiving long-term chemotherapy. Some morphologic changes in the red cells may be expected. Poikilocytosis is a common finding in dogs and cats treated with doxorubin.[125,126]

SEPSIS

Sepsis can result when the patient's own normal, motile gastrointestinal flora gain access to systemic circulation through damaged gut epithelial surfaces and proliferate during the neutropenic phase of chemotherapy. Prophylactic oral, bactericidal, broad spectrum antibiotics are indicated in patients that are afebrile and neutropenic. However, fever in a neutropenic patient is a serious finding that demands an aggressive response. Bacterial cultures of blood, urine, and any indwelling intravenous catheters should be made with appropriate sensitivity testing. Immediate treatment pending culture and sensitivity testing results should begin with intravenously administered broad spectrum, bactericidal antibiotics.

GASTROINTESTINAL TOXICITY

The spectrum of gastrointestinal toxicity following chemotherapy includes emesis, diarrhea, and anorexia. The degree of gastrointestinal toxicity varies with individual tolerance, concurrent drug administration, the degree of normal organ system compromise, and the type and dose of drug given. Gastrointestinal side effects can be very mild and transient or severe and life threatening. Fortunately most gastrointestinal side effects are mild and transient. Most of these problems can be treated symptomatically by withholding food for 24 hours and offering small amounts of bland foods such as cottage cheese and rice or a bland prescription diet when feeding is resumed. Gastrointestinal toxicity can be graded according to Table 7. Changes in dose or dosing interval may be required if toxicity is unacceptable. Remember that diarrhea accompanied by fever may be a sign of sepsis and warrents early intervention.

HEPATIC AND PANCREATIC TOXICITY

Severe hepatic toxicity associated with chemotherapy is uncommon. Sub-clinical elevations in hepatic enzymes such as SAP, GT, and ALT often follow exposure to alkylating agents. Methotrexate (an antimetabolite) has been reported to cause clinical hepatotoxicity in humans and dogs, but severe liver damage in dogs with recommended doses is rare.[127] Mild elevations in hepatic enzymes following exposure to chemotherapy are usually not clinically relevant.

Pancreatitis associated with chemotherapy is rare but has been associated with use of L-asparaginase, azathioprine, doxorubicin, epirubicin, and prednisone.[128,129] If pancreatitis is diagnosed in a patient receiving chemotherapy for cancer, treat it in the conventional manner by withholding oral food and water and by giving intravenous fluid therapy. Plasma transfusions are also indicated in cases of severe pancreatitis. Broad spectrum microbicidal antibiotics should be considered, especially if concurrent neutropenia is present. If pancreatitis occurs secondary to chemotherapy consider switching to a different drug or protocol because of the likelihood of recurrence of pancreatitis with repeated drug exposure.

CARDIOTOXICITY

The heart (dogs especially) can be adversely affected by exposure to doxorubicin and/or epirubicin.[130] These drugs are cardiotoxic secondary to free radical damage to cellular DNA and/or to topoisomerase II DNA fragmentation.[131] A safe cumulative dose range for doxorubicin administration has not unequivocally been established for dogs, but it has been established empirically as between 180 mg/m^2 and 200 mg/m^2.[120,132,133] Some dogs with cardiotoxicity from doxorubicin will develop a fatal arrhythmia and experience sudden death while others will develop congestive heart failure. Careful monitoring of total cumulative dose administered and pretreatment assessment of echocardiographic changes is vital to avoiding irreversible heart damage. Any patient being treated with doxorubicin should be assessed for ventricular systolic function by measurement of fractional shortening. This measurement is routine for monitoring of doxorubicin side effects. The ventricular fractional shorting (delta D or DD) is calculated by subtracting the end systolic dimension (ESD) from the end diastolic dimension (EDD) and dividing by the end diastolic dimension expressed as a percent (DD = EDD –ESD/EDD x 100). This calculation measures the percentage that the short axis diameter of the left ventricle shortens during systole. Fractional shortening in dogs is determined by measurements of the left ventricle made during systole and diastole at the level of the chordae tendinae and is generally accepted to be between 25% and 55% (there is considerable breed and size difference).[120] Determination of fractional short-ening should only be done by an individual with the necessary performance skill and interpretation expertise.

PULMONARY TOXICITY

Cisplatin use will cause severe pulmonary edema, hydrothorax, and mediastinal edema in cats and is contraindicated in this species.[134] Bleomycin has been reported to produce interstitial pneumonia and pulmonary fibrosis in dogs, but it is an uncommon drug in veterinary oncology.[135]

URINARY TRACT TOXICITY

Complications of chemotherapy affecting the urinary tract are usually those relating to the use of cyclophosphamide, ifosfamide, cisplatin, and corticosteroids. Of these drugs used in veterinary oncology, only cyclophosphamide and corticosteroids are truly relevant to treatment of lymphoma at this time.

Hemorrhagic cystitis will occasionally develop in patients being treated with cyclophosphamide. When it occurs, it is most commonly observed in female dogs, followed in frequency of occurrence by neutered male dogs, intact male dogs, and intact and neutered cats in about equal frequency although a recent report found no difference in risk for development of hemorrhagic cystitis with sex status.[136] This complication is attributed to the irritating effects on the bladder mucosa of a cyclophosphamide metabolite known as acrolein. Hemorrhagic cystitis can occur after prolonged drug use or after a single exposure. Secondary bacterial infection is common. The risk of hemorrhagic cystitis can be reduced by combining its use with prednisone and by giving the drug orally instead of intravenously.[136]

Studies clearly show that when cyclophosphamide is given intravenously as part of a multidrug protocol the occurrence of hemorrhagic cystitis can be reduced substantially with concurrent administration of intravenous furosemide. In a report of 216 dogs with lymphoma treated with intravenous cyclophosphamide as part of a multi-drug chemotherapy protocol, hemorrhagic cystitis developed in12 of 133 (9%) of dogs that did not receive concurrent furosemide, while only 1 of 83 dogs (1.2%) developed hemorrhagic cystitis when furosemide was given concurrently.[136]

Ifosfamide is an alkylating agent with a similar spectrum of activity to cyclophosphamide. Ifosfamide use has been reported in the treatment of dogs with lymphoma. It is expensive, requires mitigation of toxicity by using a saline diuresis and neutralization of bladder mucosa damaging metabolites with Mesna (2-mercaptoethane sulfonate), so that it is unlikely that it will find easy acceptance in veterinary oncology.

Corticosteroid use will antagonize antiduretic hormone release and activity on the distal nephron and result in decreased urine concentration, polyuria, and compensatory polydipsia. The net effect is decreased host defenses to asending infection in the urinary tract. Patients being treated with corticosteroids should be monitored for urinary tract infection.

Cisplatin is nephrotoxic, but it is not generally used in the treatment of lymphoma in dogs and its use is contraindicated in cats.[139,140] Should information regarding cisplatin administration, dose, and potential toxicity be required, consult standard reference texts.

NEUROTOXICITY

Complications of chemotherapy affecting the nervous system are usually those relating to the use of vincristine, 5-fluorouracil, and chlorambucil. Of these drugs, vincristine is the most commonly used drug in the treatment of lymphoma. 5-Fluorouracil is contraindicated in cats because of neurotoxicity concerns.[120]

Vincristine is found in many multi-drug protocols. It is very rarely associated with the development of a peripheral neuropathy that, in one canine report, was characterized by a sudden onset of shuffling of the hind paws while walking, intermittent collapse in the hind end, and difficulty in negotiationg stairs and turns. A neurologic examination of the affected dog found ataxia and depressed patellar and withdrawal reflexes in both hind limbs.

Electromyography was consistent with denervation and biopsy of a common peroneal nerve revealed a variety of myelination changes consistent with vincristine neuropathy.[141]

Chlorambucil is a nitrogen mustard derivative that acts by alkylation. It can be prescribed for use in a variety of conditions in veterinary oncology including chronic lymphocytic leukemia, low-grade lymphoma, as part of maintenance protocols for intermediate to high-grade lymphoma, mast cell tumors, multiple myeloma and to replace cyclophosphamide when sterile hemorrhagic cystitis is diagnosed. Adverse neurotoxic signs are also recognized in humans. Aldehyde metabolites of chloramubcil are thought to be responsible for the neurotoxicity. There is a hypothesis that concurrent use of corticosteroids may play a part in onset of neurotoxicity.[142]

Chlorambucil (plus prednisone) was recently reported as treatment for a cat with diffuse, low-grade intestinal lymphoma.[142] The chlorambucil was compounded in a liquid solution using a cellulose-based suspending vehicle and started at a dose of 15 mg/m^2 (4 mg total dose) daily for 4 of every 21 days. The cat was erroneously treated by the owner twice daily instead of once daily. Within 2 days the cat had neurological signs consisting of twitching and agitation that progressed to myoclonus that could be exacerbated by noise, movement, or physical restraint.

Other Treatment Options Worth Considering

RADIATION THERAPY

Lymphocytes, be they normal or malignant, are very sensitive to the effects of ionizing radiation. Most cells need to pass through cell division prior to expressing lethal radiation damage, but lymphocytes can undergo direct interphase death when exposed to clinically useful doses of radiation. Although radiation therapy has been reported to treat clinical cases of lymphoma in dogs and cats, the ideal fractionation protocol is unknown. As we discuss radiation therapy of lymphoma, it is very difficult to compare studies because of differences in the type of radiation therapy, total dose, and fractionation protocol used in the various reports. Nevertheless, the basic principal of treating lymphoma in dogs and cats with radiation therapy is well established.

Radiation therapy, at the time of this writing, is not commonly used to treat lymphoma in dogs or cats. However, when it is used, it is mostly employed to treat solitary and cutaneous tumors. Radiation therapy is also occasionally used in a palliative fashion to treat multicentric tumors that are resistant to standard chemotherapy.[143]

Dogs

Radiation therapy can also be used in a palliative manner to reduce single or regional lymph node size when the enlarged nodes are compromising the patient's quality of life. In this situation the patient is not in remission, and the goal of radiation therapy is not cure but improvement in the patient's quality of life. Mandibular and/or tracheobronchial lymphadenomegaly that cause dyspnea and/or dysphagia, or pelvic lympandenomegaly that impairs the ability to defecate are examples of situations where palliative radiation therapy may benefit the patient. Doses of 6-10 Gy often result in clinical improvement within 24 hours (the fractionation schedule will depend on the initial response to therapy and the patients status among other things).[143]

Radiation therapy has been used as the sole method of treatment for dogs with multicentric lymphoma. In one study, sequential doses of half-body radiation therapy were given to dogs 4 to 6 weeks apart. Nine of the 14 dogs in this study received the two planned half body 7 Gy doses of radiation. Of the nine dogs that received both planned treatments, 2 dogs attained a complete remission with a mean duration of remission of 101 days. Three dogs attained a partial remission with a mean duration of remission of 54 days. Serious morbidity was high among the treated dogs (acute radiation sickness in 30% of dogs after a cranial half body exposure and 80% of dogs after a caudal body exposure). Four dogs in this study died of radiation induced complications. As a result of the limited duration of remission and the high morbidity and mortality associated with this approach to treatment, radiation therapy is not recommended as the sole treatment modality for canine multicentric lymphoma.[144]

A more appropriate use of radiation therapy is for the treatment of solitary nodal and extranodal lymphoma in dogs, but these presentations are uncommon. Remember that the majority of dogs with apparent solitary disease will be found to have other sites involved or to develop more disseminated disease at a later date. For example, orthovoltage radiation therapy was reported to control lymphoma localized to the ulna and ulna-humoral joint in a 1 1/2 year old Boxer dog.[145] Three years after treatment, the dog developed multicentric lymphoma and was euthanized. Because of the high potential for systemic involvement with apparent solitary lymphoma, chemotherapy is indicated in the majority of cases.[143] Chemotherapy may be given as an adjunct to some loco-regional therapy such as surgery or radiation therapy.

Mycosis fungoides is a rare form of cutaneous lymphoma that involves T helper cells. The diagnosis of this variant of cutaneous lymphoma is based entirely on well defined histopathologic criteria with or without immunohistochemistry to confirm T cell phenotype. The use of total skin irradiation has been reported in dogs with mycosis fungoides, but too few cases have been characterized to draw conclusions regarding its efficacy.

Cats

The utility of radiation therapy in cats with lymphoma is generally limited to solitary sites that can be irridated with little systemic effect. Radiation therapy may be appropriate in cats with mediastinal lymphoma when chemotherapy must be delayed (septic patient or one with heavy bone marrow involvement). Radiation of the mediastinum has little effects on immune function compared to chemotherapy and may be used to relieve dyspnea without the risks associated with chemotherapy.[143]

Spinal lymphoma is a common non-traumatic cause of posterior paresis in cats. In most cases the lymphoma is extradural.[1,143] Chemotherapy is indicated because of the systemic nature of lymphoma. However, radiation therapy can be used to rapidly reduce tumor size and improve neurologic function.[143] Primary lymphoma of the brain is rare. However, when it occurs without systemic involvement, it is possible to treat it with radiation therapy alone. Close consultation with a medical oncologist and a radiation oncologist are advised if you encounter a patient of this nature.

Lymphoma of the nasal and paranasal sinuses is common in cats. In some surveys, nasal lymphoma is either the leading or second leading histologic malignancy type to be diagnosed in the nasal and paranasal sinuses of cats. The clinical signs of affected cats are similar to other types of tumors localized to the nasal passages. Sneezing and nasal discharge are common. Disease free interval for cats with nasal lymphoma treated with radiation therapy can be 1-2 years. Cats with clinical stage I or II have a better prognosis than cats with more disseminated disease.[143] It is unclear whether concurrent chemotherapy is needed for cats with nasal lymphoma that receive radiation therapy as primary therapy. However, the limited data available suggest that chemotherapy as an adjunct to radiation therapy offers a survival advantage because of the potential for occult and concurrent systemic involvement of lymphoma.[143]

Mycosis fungoides is very rare in cats, but radiation therapy may be useful in the treatment of cutaneous lymphoma in cats that occur as solitary lesions that are not amenable to complete surgical removal. As in other cases of apparent solitary localization of disease, concurrent chemotherapy is advised.

CHEMOTHERAPY COMBINED WITH RADIATION THERAPY

Radiation therapy can be used in combination with chemotherapy to treat multicentric disease when single or regional lymph nodes have not responded completely to induction chemotherapy. In the second situation, radiation theapy can used in an attempt to induce a complete remission when disease is undetectable at other sites.

There are a few recent reports of chemotherapy being combined with half-body radiation therapy.[146-148] In general the patient is first treated with chemotherapy to achieve a complete remission, and this is followed by treatment with half-body irridation (either the cranial or caudal half with the zyphoid as the dividing point). For example, one study of 50 dogs with lymphoma were treated by inducing remission with chemotherapy over 11 weeks (prednisone, L-asparaginase, vincristine, doxorubicin, cyclophosphamide) followed by first cranial half-body radiation then three weeks later caudal half-body radiation therapy. Radiation was administered at a dose of 8Gy per half-body given in 2 consecutive 4Gy fractions. For the 34 dogs that achieved complete remission, the median first remission duration was 201 days.[149]

Nutritional Therapy

Cancer, including lymphoma, can cause a variety of effects that affect host metabolism. It is well established that dogs with lymphoma have abnormal carbohydrate metabolism (hyperlactatemia and hyperinsulinemia) that remains uncorrected even after successful clinical remission with chemotherapy.[150] Altered carbohydrate metabolism is a part of the mechanisms for cachexia in some cancer patients.

Polyunsaturated n-3 fatty acids have been shown to inhibit growth and metastasis of tumors. In addition, several amino acids are important in the nutritional treatment discussion of cancer patients. For example, arginine has been shown to decrease tumor growth and metastatic rate in rodent cancer models. The mechanism of this benefit is unclear, but arginine given to mature, healthy dogs has been shown to be a secretagogue for growth hormone that can regenerate the normally atrophied thymus glands in theses dogs with some potential for immune enhancement.[151]

One study tested the hypothesis that nutritional intervention may extend the disease free interval and survival time for dogs with lymphoma. Thirty two dogs with stage IIIa or IVa lymphoma were randomized to receive doxorubicin chemotherapy plus a diet supplemented with fish oil (rich in polyunsaturated n-3 fatty acids) and arginine, or the same chemotherapy plus the same diet supplemented with soybean oil. The median disease free interval for dogs getting the fish oil and arginine supplementation was 209 days versus 144 days for the control group. The median survival for the dogs getting fish oil and arginine supplementation was 319 days versus 232 days for the control group. The dogs on the experimental diet had normalization of elevated blood lactic acid in a dose dependent manner. The authors of this study concluded that the normalization of lactate resulted in an increase in the disease free interval and survival for dogs with lymphoma.[152] The results of this study became the basis for the prescription diet n/d®*.

Rescue Therapy

At some point in the course of treatment, the vast majority of patients will become resistant to chemotherapy. In response to this basic principal, thoughtful clinicians will develop rescue plans early in the decision making process. Rescue implies that resistance to the primary or subsequent drug protocol has happened, that the patient maintains the necessary physical reserves for additional treatment, and the owner has the endurance and resources (emotional and financial) to continue. Because resistance to the primary protocol has occurred, it is very likely that subsequent remissions will be progressively shorter in duration until nothing is effective. At this point the disease becomes insurmountable, and the patient will die or be euthanatized. Drugs that have been used for rescue therapy for dogs with lymphoma include doxorubicin, mitoxantrone, actinomycin D, etoposide, mechlorethamine, imidazone carboxamide, cisplatin, cytosine arabinoside, plus others alone or in combination.[147,153] All of these agents have some drawbacks including high purchase price, laborious administration, and/or potentially hazardous exposure to health care professionals that prepare and/or administer them. Rescue protocols result in 10-40% complete response rates with duration of remission ranging from 1 to 5 months.[153] Little has been published about specific rescue therapy for cats with lymphoma.

* Hill's Pet Nutrition, Topeka, KS

Doxorubicin alone can be an effective rescue for dogs that have previously been treated with a non-doxorubicin containing protocol such as COP. Likewise, COP can be an effective rescue plan for dogs first treated with doxorubicin alone. In one study where 11 of 43 dogs with lymphoma previously treated with doxorubicin alone, 6 dogs attained a CR and 2 attained a PR (3 dogs were lost to follow up or declined additional treatment) when subsequently treated with COP. The median duration remission of the 8 dogs with adequate follow-up was 104 days (range; 43-148 days).[154]

Doxorubicin (30 mg/m^2 IV on day one) plus dacarbazine (200 mg/^{2} IV once daily on days 1 through 5) induced a second complete remission in 5 of 15 dogs with lymphoma that were resistant to doxorubicin alone. Three additional dogs had a partial remission in response to this treatment. The median survival time for the 5 dogs that completely responded was 105 days (range, 45-241 days). Treatment resulted in a severe neutropenia in three dogs with one death attributed to sepsis.[155]

Mitoxantrone given at 6mg/m^2 IV to dogs with lymphoma after the first relapse resulted in complete response in 7 of 15 dogs (47%) with a median duration of response in the 7 dogs of 84 days. Toxicities were mild. Nine of 15 dogs (60%) attained a complete remission with additional chemotherapy after failing mitoxantrone treatment.[156]

Cytosine arabinoside is an antimetabolite drug that has not been effective as an induction agent when used alone at standard doses. Limited personal experience suggests that it can be safely used as a rescue agent for dogs with resistant lymphoma when given at 600 mg/m^2 IV once a week; however duration of response is short.

Two different studies have been published that evaluated the effectiveness of actinomycinD as a rescue agent for dogs with resisitant lymphoma. However, the studies yielded dramatically different results. In the first study, 9 of 12 dogs with resistant lymphoma responded to 0.5 to 0.7 mg/m^2 IV of actinomycin D give every three weeks.[157] Of the 9 dogs that responded, only three had previously been exposed to doxorubicin and 5 had complete remissions (median duration of remission was 63 days) and 4 had partial remissions (median duration of 31.5 days).[157] The second sudy of 25 dogs with resistant lymphoma that were treated with a median dose of actinomycin D of 0.7 mg/m^2 IV every three weeks failed to induce remission in any of the dogs.[158] Because 23 of the 25 dogs in this later study had prior treatment that included doxorubicin, the authors speculate that P-glycoprotein multi-drug resistance (confirmed in 2 dogs) was responsible for this failure.[158]

Lomustine is currently the rescue drug of choice for multi-drug protocol resistant lymphoma. In one study of 43 dogs that failed previous chemotherapy, a complete response to lomustine was observed in 3 dogs with a median duration of response of 110 days (range; 60 to 212 days).[159] A partial response to lomustine was observed in an additional 8 dogs with a median response duration of 75 days (range; 36 to 211 days). The doses of lomustine used in this study ranged from 90–100 mg/m^2 orally every three weeks.

A more recent retrospective study of lomustine (dose range of 60-90 mg/m^2) as a first rescue agent for 38 dogs resistant to the University of Wisconsin-Madison protocol resulted in a response rate of 59% (18% CR). Median duration of remission was not given. Grade 3 hematologic toxicity in either neutrophils or platelets was observed in 9.5% of dogs and grade 4 hematologic toxicity was observed in 25% of dogs.[160]

Another small study of lomustine given at even lower doses (50-70 mg/m^2 every 21 days) as rescue to 9 dogs resistant to COPLA failed to significantly prolong disease in most dogs in the study. Although the response rate was 66%, the median duration of remission was only 21 days. It appears that higher doses of lomustine are necessary for lomustine to be considered an appropriate rescue agent despite the increased risks of toxicity.[161]

Myelosuppression from lomustine can be severe and much lower doses are now recommended than were used in early studies. A more appropriate dose of lomustine given orally every three weeks is 70 mg/m^2, but if the patient fails to tolerate that dose subsequent doses can be as low as 50 mg/m^2.[162] Suggested rescue protocols are given in Table 16.

TABLE 16

RESCUE PROTOCOLS FOR DOGS WITH LYMPHOMA

Number of Animals	Overall Response (%)	Complete Response (%)	Median Duration of Response (days)	Median Duration of Complete Response (days)
Actinomycin-D				
12	66	42	42	63

Comments

Potentially useful if doxorubicin has not been previously used. A confirmatory study is needed. See text.
Suggested dose is 0.6 mg/^{2} IV every 21 days.[153]

Actinomycin-D				
25	---	---	---	---

Comments

Not effective in patients that have previously been treated with doxorubicin. See text. Suggested dose is 0.6 mg/^{2} IV every 21 days.[154]

Doxorubicin				
---	----	----	----	----

Comments

Of use if no prior treatment with doxorubicin

Doxorubicin plus dacarbazine				
15	53	33	<42	Not reported

Comments

Fairly toxic to bone marrow. Doxorubicin, 30mg/m^2 or 1 mg/kg for dogs under 10 kg body weight on day 1 plus dacarbazine, 200mg/m^2 as a slow IV bolus once daily on days 1-5. Use concurrent antiemetics like metoclopraminde on days 1-5. Repeat every 21 days.[151]

Mitoxantrone				
44	41	30	Not reported	127

Comments

Well tolerated. Use Mitoxantrone at 6mg/m^2 IV every 21 days.[152]

Lomustine				
43	25	7	Not reported	110

Use 50-70 mg/m^2 orally every three weeks.[155]

Cytosine arabinoside				
---	---	----	---	----

Comments

600 mg/m^2 IV each week

2)

Cutaneous
Lymphoma

Lymphoma involving the skin in dogs and cats is relatively uncommon. Cutaneous lymphoma accounts for 3%-8% of all cases of lymphosarcoma reported in dogs.[163,164]   Reliable information on occurrence rates in cats is unavailable, but in general, it is safe to conclude that cutaneous lymphoma occurs less frequently in cats than in dogs. This form of lymphoma tends to occur in older animals with a mean age of onset in dogs of 9.5 years and 11 years in cats.[165-167] In several studies of cats with this form of lymphoma, all cats tested were FeLV test negative.[165-169] Cutaneous lymphoma can occur as the primary form, or it may disseminate to or from other areas.

Cutaneous lymphoma is usually categorized as being either epitheliotrophic (epidermotrophic) which tend to consist of a population of T-cells, or nonepitheiotrophic which tends to consist of B-cells or occasionally null cells (not classifiable as either B-cells or T-cells).[163,164-170]

Epitheliotrophic cutaneous lymphoma can be subdivided into three forms: mycosis fungoides, Sézary syndrome, or pagetoid reticulosis. Of these subtypes, mycosis fungoides is the most common among dogs and cats.[163,171]

Mycosis fungoides is a non-leukemic variant of cutaneous lymphoma that is reported occasionally in dogs, but rarely in cats (Figure 18A and B). In dogs the neoplastic cells involved are thought to be memory T-cells and stain CD8+. It is characterized histologically by lymphocyte infiltration of the skin, minimal spongiosis, and Pautrier's microablcesses (a discrete accmulation of neoplastic cells in the epidermis) that are characteristic histologic features of mycosis fungoides.[163,166,170]

Sézary syndrome or Sézary-like disease is reported in both dogs and cats. It is characterized by the presence of cutaneous lymphoma (generalized, exfoliative erythroderma and lymphadenomegaly) plus leukemia. Pruritus is common. Histologic assessment of skin biopsy specimens is consistent with that of mycosis fungoides, but it has the additional feature of having circulating neoplastic lymphocytes

FIGURE 18A

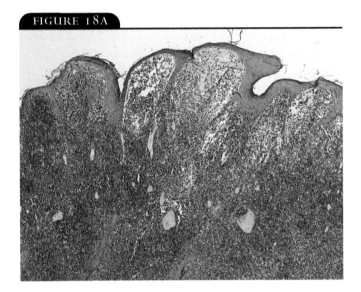

FIGURE 18B

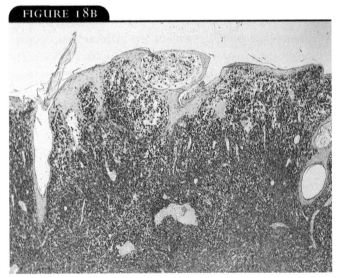

A. Mycosis Fungoides, H&E x 500. Skin of a 12 year old spayed female domestic cat that presented for apparent pruritus with swelling, redness, and hair loss at the tip of the tail. A biopsy revealed a solid proliferation of lymphocytes that has infiltrated the superficial and deep dermis forming pockets of lymphoid infiltration into the epidermis. (Pautrier's microabscess, top center of image). (Courtesy of Dr. Ted Valli.)
B. Mycosis Fungoides, CD3 x 500. The same lesion as described in figure 18A showing positive CD3 staining indicating the presence of T-lymphocytes. (Courtesy of Dr. Ted Valli.)

that appear as large, convoluted cells with hyperchromatic nuclei and a high nuclear:cytoplasmic ratio that are known as Sézary cells. [163,169,171]

Pagetoid reticulosis can resemble mycosis fungoides and Sézary syndrome histologically because it has the feature of a monomorphus population of neoplastic lymphoid cells infiltrating the epidermis (Figures 19A and B). However, it is reported to take a relatively benign course as a solitary plaque of chronic duration.[172]

Histologically B-cell non-epitheliotrophic lymphoma is characterized by localization of malignant lymphocytes located deeper in the dermis with sparing of the papillary dermis and epidermis. The neoplastic cell population of this form has been classified in the literature as being well differentiated, poorly differentiated, undifferentiated, or large cell. Because T-cell lymphoma can also appear as a non-epitheiotrophic form, the lack of epidermal infiltration by lymphocytes is not a useful criterion in defining B-cell or T-cell variants of this disorder. Immunhistochemistry plus routine histologic assessment can be used to distinguish B-cell from T-cell lymphoma. Lesions are usually discrete solitary or multifocal nodules that may have an acute onset and rapid progression.[163,166-173]

FIGURE 19A

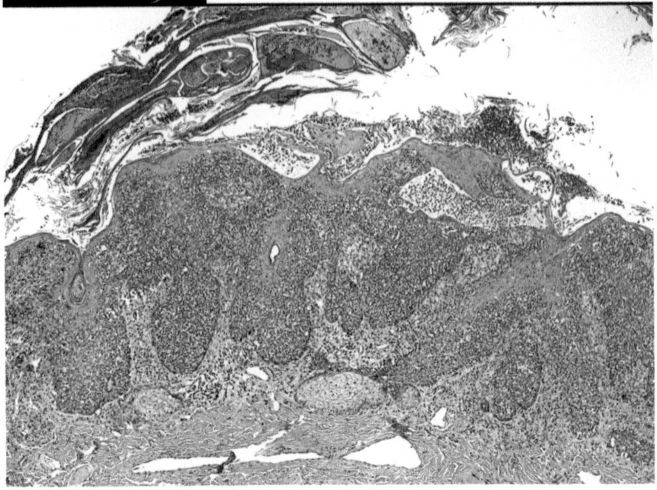

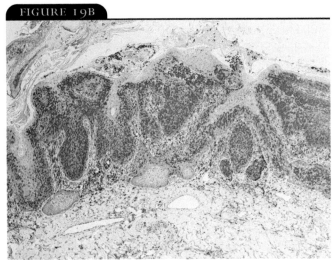

FIGURE 19B

A. Pagetoid Reticulosis, H&E x 500. Gingiva of a 10 year old spayed female coon hound dog that presented for a persistent swelling. A biopsy revealed marked thickening of the epidermis, superficial crusting, and formation of large irregular-shaped rete pegs that have a very heavy cellular infiltration. There is a much less dense cellular infiltration into the surrounding superficial dermis with the deep dermal tissues largely uninvolved. (Courtesy of Dr. Ted Valli.)
B. Pagetoid Reticulosis, CD3 x 500. The same lesion as described in figure 19A but showing strong and uniform positive staining for CD3. Note that CD3 positive staining is largely confined to the epithelium with only scattered labeling of the cells in the superficial dermis. The skin glands and deeper dermis are spared. (Courtesy of Dr. Ted Valli.)

Clinical Features

Lesions of cutaneous lymphoma, regardless of subtype, typically occur as single or multifocal lesions on any skin surface, but it often includes mucocutaneous and/or oral cavity involvement. Cutaneous lymphoma can progress through stages of exfoliative erythroderma, plaque formation, and nodule formation, or present as nodular disease from the outset. Lesions may also resemble pustules or be depigmented. The size of the involved areas can be small (few millimeters) or large nodules or plaques (centimeters in diameter).[163,166,169-173]

Some animals may initially have coalescing, erythematous patches with alopecia and scale on the head and face that progress to the trunk. This initial lesion may progress to circular then irregular ehrthemic plaques, some with central ulceration, and dry crusts at mucocutaneous junctions. Plaque formation is more common in cats than dogs. Pruritus is variable with patch and plaque forms, but cats tend to be more pruritic than dogs and may show more self-trauma and ulceration.[163] Both patch and plaque forms can regress and reappear at a later date or progress rapidly to a more aggressive cutaneous malignancy.

Variable sized, painless solitary or multiple nodules can appear as firm, elevated, dark red, shiny, scaly, or ulcerated lesions with serous oozing onto the skin surface. Exudate can form a crust on top of the nodule. The combination of ulcerative skin disease with crusting can lead to areas of matted hair with a foul odor. Secondary bacterial infection can exacerbate pruritus. Spread to lymph nodes or other organs can occur.[163,166]

Because of its variable clinical presentation, misdiagnosing cutaneous lymphoma is easy and common. Patients may present for a second opinion after many months of therapy in which antibiotics, dips, and corticosteroids were not successful in curing the misdiagnosed problem. In one study of cutaneous lymphoma, 64% (14/22) of dogs presented with a history of chronic dermatitis.[167]

The various manifestations of cutaneous lymphoma in dogs have been misdiagnosed as endocrine alopecia, seborrhea, atopic dermatitis, pododermatitis, or pyoderma. In cats, differential diagnosis should include dermatophytosis, allergic dermatitis, eosinophilic plaque formation, autoimmune skin disorders, drug eruptions and ectoparasites (especially Cheyletiella).[163,166,168]

DOGS

In one report of 26 dogs with epitheliotrophic cutaneous lymphoma, 80% had erythema at presentation, 57% had plaques, and 62% had scales.[166] Mucosal lesions are reported to occur in one third of affected dogs.[166]

CATS

Overall, the progression of cutaneous lymphoma in cats appears to be similar to dogs (patch, plaque, then nodular). In a retrospective study of nine cats with cutaneous lymphoma, 5 cats had solitary masses, 4 had multiple or diffuse lesions, and 1 was classified as mycosis fungoides.[165]

Diagnosis and Staging

The diagnosis of cutaneous lymphoma is established with biopsy. Although a fine needle aspiration biopsy is adequate for diagnosis, histologic assessment is essential for full characterization of the disorder. Every effort should be made to clearly establish the tumor as either B-cell origin or T-cell origin. Staging of cutaneous lymphoma is the same as for other forms.

Treatment and Prognosis

Treatment of cutaneous lymphoma is often frustrating and disappointing. Many treatment modalities must be considered merely palliative, but some relief from clinical symptoms can often be offered. For example, regular bathing with soothing shampoos may increase comfort and appearance, but they have no effect on the primary disease. Prednisone can be used successfully to control pruritus, but probably has no appreciable effect on survival.

Traditional and non-traditional modalities of treatment can be employed to treat dogs and cats with cutaneous lymphoma.

Surgery has been reported to be effective primary therapy in some dogs with cutaneous lymphoma. In one report of 22 dogs with cutaneous lymphoma, 8 had solitary lesions and 7 of these were treated by surgical excision. Of the dogs treated by surgery, 4 were considered by the authors to be "cured."[166] Cats may be more difficult to successfully treat with surgery alone.

Radiation therapy has been utilized to treat solitary or multifocal lesions. Dogs with mycosis fungoides can have healing and regression of lesions following treatment with radiation therapy.[175,177]

A variety of chemotherapy protocols have been used to treat cutaneous lymphoma in dogs and cats.[165-167,170,174] The use of topical nitrogen mustard (mechlorethamine) was reported effective in some dogs, but it has a high incidence of allergic and irritant contact sensitization in people exposed to it. Cats tend to have significant bone marrow suppression and gastrointestinal upset when treated with nitrogen mustard.[169]

The best survival times for cutaneous lymphoma are usually the result of treatment with combination chemotherapy protocols, especially those containing doxorubicin. Remission of 46 days was reported in one dog with epitheliotrophic cutaneous lymphoma treated with chlorambucil and prednisone , while a remission of 304 days was reported in another dog treated with doxorubicin, vincrisitine, and prednisone.[166]

Retinoids have gained a secure place in the treatment of cutaneous lymphoma. The exact mode of action of retinoids on neoplastic lymphocytes is unknown. Because retinoids are a vitamin A analog and vitamin A helps to regulate growth and differentiation of cells, retinoids may act by regulating epithelial differentiation and reversing malignant differentiation. In one report of retinoid treatment of 14 dogs with cutaneous lymphoma, clinical remission (greater or equal to 50% reduction in erythema, scaling, or pruritus for at least 4 months) was observed in 6 of the dogs.[172] Twelve dogs were treated with isotretinoin and 2 were treated with etretinate. Of the 12 dogs with epitheliotrophic lymphoma treated with isotretinoin, 4 responded for between 152 and 395 days. One of the dogs responded to etretinate for 456 days, while one dog with nonepitheliotrophic cutaneous lymphoma responded to isotretinoin for 535 days. For all dogs in this study with epitheliotrophic lymphoma, the mean remission/survival was 328 days. The study authors recommended a dose of 3-4 mg/kg of isotretinoin each day for treatment of cutaneous lymphoma.[172] Side effects of isotretinoin in dogs included panting, salivation, mild dry cough, corneal lipid deposits, and high serum triglyceride values. Side effects in dogs treated with etretinate included abdominal alopecia. Adverse effects of retinoid therapy did not correlate with dose and occurred only sporadically. Most abnormalities were transient and reversible upon cessation of therapy.[172] Other infrequent adverse side effects reported for retinoids include keratoconjunctivitis sicca, swollen tongue, polydipsia, signs of joint pain, pruritus, hyperlipidemia, hyperactivity, ear pruritus, erhtyema of the feet and mucocutaneous junctions, lethargy or anorexia with vomiting, and teratogenesis.[176,177]

Of 3 cats with epitheliotrophic lymphoma treated with isotretinoin (10mg daily), all had a good clinical response and showed reduction of erythema and scaling with re-growth of hair. Complete remission was not attained in any of the cats.[177]

In a separate study of 3 cats with epitheliotrophic lymphoma treated with 1 mg/kg of isotretinoin every 12-24 hours, some improvement of clinical symptoms were observed, but no complete remissions were documented.[163] Survival in this study ranged from 182-547 days. Diarrhea was the only side effect noted in 1 cat treated with isotretinoin. Other side effects noted sporadically in cats given isotretinoin include periocular edema, periocular crusting, epiphora, and plepharospasm.[168]

References

1. Vonderhaar MA, Morrison WB. Lymphosarcoma. In: Morrison WB (ed). Cancer in Dogs and Cats : Medical and Surgical Management, 2nd ed. Jackson, WY: Teton NewMedia 2002:641-670.

2. Dorn CR, Taylor DO, Hibbard HH. Epizootiologic characteristics of canine and feline leukemia and lymphosarcoma. Am J Vet Res. 1967;28: 993-1001.

3. Ipsos Marketing Research, New York, NY 2002

4. Teske E, van Straten G, van Noort R, Rutteman GR. Chemotherapy with cyclophosphamide, vincristine, and pred-nisolone (COP) in cats with malignant lymphoma: New results with an old protocol. J Vet Int Med 2002;16:179-186.

5. Romantowski J, Lubkin SR. Use of an epidemologic model to evaluate feline leukemia virus control measures. Feline Pract 1997;25:6-11.

6. Hayes HM, Tarone RE, Cantor KP, et al. Case control study of canine malignant lymphosarcoma: Positive association with dog owners use of 2,4-dichlorophenoxyacetic acid herbicides. J Natl Cancer Inst 1991:83; 1226-1231. JNCI 1991:83;1226-31.

7. Reif JS, Lower KS, Ogilvie GK. Residential exposure to magnetic fields and risk of canine lymphosarcoma. Am J Epidemiol 1995:141; 352-359.

8. Hahn KA, Richardson RC, Hahn EA, Chrisman CL. Diagnostic and prognostic importance of chromosomal aberrations identified in 61 dogs with lymphosarcoma. Vet Pathol 1994;31:528-540.

9. Chaganti SR, Mitra J, LoBue J. Detection of canine homologs of human MYC, BCL2, IGH, and TCRB genes by Southern blot analysis. Cancer Genet Cytogenet 1992;62:9-14.

10. Edwards MD, Pazzi KA, Gumerlock PH, et al. c-N-ras is activated infrequently in canine malignant lymphoma. Toxicol Pathol 1993;21:288-291.

10a. Gabor LJ, Jackson ML, Trask B, Malik R, Canfield PJ. Feline leukaemia virus status of Australian cats with lymphosarcoma. Aust Vet J 2001;79:476-481.

10b. Davidson EB, Gregory CR, Kass PH. Surgical excision of soft tissue fibrosarcomas in cats. Vet Surg 1997;26:265-269.

10c. Madewell BR, Gieger TL, Pesavento PA, Kent MS. Vaccine site-associated sarcoma and malignant lymphoma in cats: a report of six cases (1997-2002). J Am Anim Hosp Assoc 2004; 40:47-50.

11. Barr MC, Olsen CW, Scott FW. Feline viral diseases. In: Ettinger SJ, Feldman EC (eds): Textbook of Veterinary Internal Medicine. Philadelphia, WB Saunders, 1995; 4th edition, 409-439.

12. Vobis M, D'Haese J, Melhorn H, Mencke N. The feline leukemia virus (FeLV) and the cat flea (Centocephalides felis). Parasitol Res 2003;90:S132-S134.

13. Richards J, Rodan I, Elston T, Flemming D, Ford R, Henry S, Hustead D, Lappin M, Paul M, Rosen D, Scherk M, Scott F, Welborn L. 2000 Report of the American Association of Feline Practitioners and the Academy of Feline Medicine Advisory Panel on Feline Vaccines. AAFP, 2000.

14. Herring ES, Troy GC, Toth TE, Forrester SD, Weigt LA, Herring IP. Detection of feline leukemia virus in blood and bone marrow of cats with varying suspicion of latent infection. J Feline Med and Surg 2001;3:133-141.

15. Morrison WB. The new language of oncology: terms used in molecular biology relating to cancer In: Morrison WB (ed). Cancer in Dogs and Cats: Medical and Surgical Management, 2nd ed. Jackson, WY: Teton NewMedia 2002:13-8.

16. Rosenthal N. DNA and the genetic code. New Engl J Med 1994;331:39-41.

17. Morrison, WB, Starr RM, Vaccine-Associated Feline Sarcoma Task Force. Vaccine-associated feline sarcomas. J Am Vet Med Assoc 2001;218:697-699.

18. Valli VE, Jacobs RM, Parodi AL, Vernau W, Moore PF. Histologic classification of hematopoietic tumors of domestic animals. Washington DC. Armed Forces Institute of Pathology and World Health Organization collaborating Center for Worldwide References on Comparative Oncology 2002.

19. Valli VE, Jacobs R, Norris A, Couto C, Morrison W, McCaw D, Cotter S, Ogilvie G, Moore A. The histological classification of 602 cases of feline lymphoporliferative diseases using the national cancer institute working formulation. J Vet Diagn Invest 2000;12:295-306.

20. Carter RF, Valli VEO, Lumsden JH. The cytology, histology and prevalence of cell types in canine lymphosarcoma classified according to the national cancer institute working formulation. Can J Vet Res. 1986;50:154-164.

21. Teske E. Canine malignant lymphosarcoma: A review and comparison with human non-Hodgkin's lymphosarcoma. Vet Quarterly. 1994(16); 4:209-19.

22. Teske E, van Heerd P, Rutteman GR, Kurzman ID, Moore PF, MacEwen EG. Prognostic factors for treatment of malignant lymphoma in dogs. J Am Vet Med Assoc1994;205:1722-1728.

23. Kiupel M, Teske E, Bostock D. Prognostic factors for treated canine malignant lymphoma. Vet Pathol 1999;36:292-300.

24. Rushlander DM, Gebhard DH, Tompkins MB, Grindem CB, Page RL. Immunophenotypic characterization of canine lymphoprolifera-tive disorders. In Vivo 1997;11:169-172.

25. Day MJ. Immunophenotypic characterization of cutaneous lymphoid neoplasia in the dog and cat. J Comp Pathol 1995;112:79-96.

26. Greenlee PG, Filippa DA, Quimby FW, et al. Lymphosarcomas in dogs, a morphologic, immunologic and clinical study. Cancer 1990;66:480-490.

27. Aquino SM, Hamor RE, Valli VE, Kitchell BE, Tunev SS, Bailey KL, Ehrart EJ. Progression of an orbital T-cell rich B-cell lymphoma to B-cell lymphoma in a dog. Vet Pathol 2000;37:465-469.

28. Steele KE, Saunders GK, Coleman GD. T-cell-rich B-cell lymphoma in a cat. Vet Pathol 1997;34:47-49.

29. Day MJ, Kyaw-Tanner M, Silkstone MA, Lucke VM, Robinson WF. T-cell-rich B-cell lymphoma in the cat. J Comp Path 1999;120:155-167.

30. Rassnick KM, Moroff SD, Mauldin GN. Prognostic value of AgNORs in feline intestinal lymphoma. Proceedings of the Veterinary Cancer Society (abstract) 1995;15:13.

31. Vail DM, Kisselberth WC, Obradovich JE, Moore FM, London CA, MacEwen EG, Ritter MA. Assessment of potential doubling time (Tpot), argyrophilic nucleolar organizer regions, (AgNOR), and proliferating cell nuclear antigen (PCNA) as predictors of therapy response in canine non-Hodgkin's lymphoma. Int Soc Exp Hematol 1996;24:807-815.

32. Vail DM, Kravis LD, Kisseberth WC, et al. FNA determination of AgNOR and CD3 status from dogs with LSA. In: Veterinary Cancer Society 15th Annual Conference Proceedings (abstract). 1995;56.

33. Johnson GC, Miller MA, Ramos-Vara JA. Comparisons of argyrophilic nucleolar organizer regions (AgNORs) and mitotic index in distinguishing benign from malignant canine smooth muscle tumors and in separating inflammatory hyperplasia from neoplastic lesions of the urinary bladder mucosa. J Vet Diagn Invest 1995;7:127-136.

34. Kravis LD, Vail DM, Kisselberth WC, Ogilvie GK, Volk LM. Frequency of argyrophilic nucleolar organizer regions in fine-needle aspirates and biopsy specimens from mast cell tumors in dogs. J Am Vet Med Assoc 1996;209:1418-1420.

35. Carter RF. Cell types in canine lymphosarcoma: Morphology, morphometry, phenotypes and prognostic correlations. Guelph, Ontario, Canada: The University of Guelph; 1987. Thesis.

36. Madewell BR, Theilen GH. Hematopoietic neoplasms, sarcomas and related conditions: Canine. Part IV. In: Theilen GH, Madewell BR, eds. Veterinary Cancer Medicine, 2nd ed. Philadelphia, PA: Lea & Febiger; 1987:392-407.

37. Leifert CE, Matus RE. Canine lymphosarcoma: clinical considerations. Semin Vet Med/Surg (Sm Anim). 1986;1:43-50.

38. Couto CG. Canine Lymphosarcomas: Something old, something new. Comp Cont Ed. 1985;7:291-302.

39. Cotter SM, Goldstein MA. Comparison of two protocols for maintenance of remission in dogs with lymphosarcoma. J Am Anim Hosp Assoc. 1987;23:495-499.

40. MacEwen EG, Young KM. Canine lymphosarcoma and lymphoid leukemias. In: Small Animal Clinical Oncology, 2nd ed. Withrow SJ and MacEwen EG (eds). WB Saunders Company, Philadelphia, 1996: 451-479.

41. Ogilvie GK, Moore AS. Lymphosarcoma. In: Managing the veterinary cancer patient. Veterinary Learning Systems Co., Inc., Trenton, 1995: 228-259.

42. Ogilvie GK, Moore AS. Lymphosarcoma. In: Managing the veterinary cancer patient. Veterinary Learning Systems Co, Inc., Trenton, 1995: 249-259.

43. Mooney SC, AK, Hayes AA, MacEwen EG. Generalized lymphadenopathy resembling lymphosarcoma in cats: Six cases (1972-1976). J Amer Vet Med Assoc 1987; 190:897-900.

44. McDonnough SP, Van Winkle TJ, Valentine BA, vanGessel YA, Summers BA. Clinicopathological and immunophenotypical features of canine intravascular lymphoma (malignant angioendotheliomatosis). Proceedings of the Veterinary Cancer Society Mid-Year Conference (abstract) 2002, 28.

44a. Fry MM, Vernau W, Pesavento PA, Brömel C, Moore PF. Hepatospleinic lymphoma in a dog. Vet Pathol 2003; 40:556-562.

45. Savary KCM, Price GS, Vaden SL. Hypercalcemia in cats: a retrospective study of 71 cases (1991-1997). J Vet Int Med 2000;14:184-189.

46. Carreras JK, Goldschmidt M, Lamb M, McLear RC, Drobatz KJ, Søremo KU. Feline epitieliotrophic intestinal malignant lymphoma: 10 cases (1997-2000). J Vet Intern Med 2003;17:326-331.

47. Mahony OM, Moore AS, Cotter SM, et al. Alimentary lymphoma in cats 28 cases (1988-1993). J Am Vet Med Assoc 1995;207:1593-1598.

48. French RA, Seitz SE, Valli VEO. Primary epitheliotrophic alimentary T-cell lymphoma with hepatic involvement in a dog. Vet Pathol 1996;33:349352.

49. Fondacaro JV, Richter KP, Carpenter JL, et al. Feline gastrointestinal lymphoma:67 cases (1988-1996). Eur J Comp Gastrointerol 1999;4:5-11.

50. Krecic MR, Black SS. Epitheliotrophic T-cell gastrointestinal tract lymphosarcoma with metastases to lung and skeletal muscle in a cat. J Am Vet Med Assoc 2000;216:524-529.

51. Wellman ML, Hammer AS, DiBartola SP, et al. Lymphosarcoma involving large granular lymphocytes in cats: 11 cases (1982-1991). J Amer Vet Med Assoc 1992; 210:1265-1269.

52. Darbès J, Majzoub M, Breuer W, Hermanns W. Large granular lymphocyte leukemia/lymphoma in six cats. Vet Pathol 1998;35:370-379.

53. Callanan JJ, Jones BA, Irvine J. Histologic classification and immunophenotype of lymphosarcomas in cats with naturally and experimentally acquired feline immunodeficiency virus infections. Vet Pathol 1996;33:264-272.

54. McMillan FD. Hypercalcemia associated with lymphoid neoplasia in two cats. Feline Pract 1985; 15:31-4.

55. Klein MK. Personal communication.

56. Weller RE, Stann SE. Renal lymphosarcoma in the cat. J Amer Anim Hosp Assoc 1983;19:363.

57. Mooney S, Hayes A, Matus R, et al. Renal lymphosarcoma in cats: 28 cases (1977-1984) J Am Vet Med Assoc 1987; 191:1473-77.

58. Carpenter JL, Andrews LK, Holzworth J. Tumors and tumor-like lesions. In: Holzworth J, (ed). Diseases of the Cat: Medicine and Surgery. WB Saunders, Philadelphia, 1987:406-597.

59. Swanson JF. Ocular manifestations of systemic disease. Vet Clin North Am, Small Anim Prac 1990; 20:849-67.

60. Parnell NK, Powell, LL, Hohenhaus AE, Patnaik AK, Peterson ME. Hypoadrenocorticism as the primary manifestation of lymphoma in two cats. J Am Vet Med Assoc 1999;214:1208-1211.

61. Madewell BR. Hematologic and bone marrow cytological abnormalities in 75 dogs with malignant lymphosarcoma. J Am Anim Hosp Assoc 1986; 22:235-40.

62. Ogilvie GK, Moore AS. Paraneoplastic syndromes. In: Managing the veterinary cancer patient. Veterinary Learning Systems Co, Inc., Trenton, 1995: 197-222.

63. Ruslander D, Page R. Perioperative management of paraneoplastic syndromes. In: The Veterinary Clinics of North America, Small Animal Practice-Surgical Oncology. Gilson SD, ed. WB Saunders Company, Philadelphia; 1995:25:1:47-62.K

64. Kissebirth WC, MacEwen EG. Complications of cancer and its treatment. In: Small Animal Clinical Oncology. 2nd edition. Withrow SJ and MacEwen EG (eds). WB Saunders Company, Philadelphia, 1996: 129-146.

65. Raskin RE, Krehbiel JD. Prevalence of leukemic blood and bone marrow in dogs with multicentric lymphosarcoma. J Am Vet Med Assoc. 1989;194:1427-1429.

66. Hardy WD. Hematopoietic tumors of cats. J Amer Anim Hosp Assoc 1981; 17:921-940.

67. Couto CG. Oncology. In: The Cat: Diseases and Clinical Management. Sherding RG (ed). Churchill Livingstone, New York, 1989:589-647.

68. Jordan HL, Grindem CB, Breitschwerdt EB. Thrombocytopenia in cats: A retrospective study in 41 cases. J Vet Intern Med 1993; 7:261-265.

69. Spodnick GJ, Berg J, Moore FM, Cotter SM. Spinal lymphosarcoma in cats : 21 cases (1976-1989). 1992; 200:373-376.

70. Williams DA, Goldschmidt MH. Hyperviscosity syndrome with IgM monoclonal gammopathy and hepatic plasmacytoid lymphosarcoma in a cat. J Small Anim Prac 1982; 23:311.

70a. Kadar E, Rush JE, Wetmore, L, Chan DL. Electrolyte disturbances and cardiac arrhythmias in a dog following pamidronate, calcitonin, and furosemide administration for hypercalcemia of malignancy. J Am Anim Hosp Assoc 2004;40:75-81.

70b. Rambeiha WL, Kruger JM, Fitzgerald SF, Nachreiner RF, Kaneene JB, Braselton WE, Chiapuzio Cl. Use of pamidronate to reverse vitamin D_3-induced toxicosis in dogs. Am J Vet Res 1999;60:1092-1097.

71. Morrison WB. Paraneoplastic syndromes and the tumors that cause them. In: Morrison WB (ed). Cancer in Dogs and Cats: Medical and Surgical Management, 2nd ed. Jackson, WY: Teton NewMedia 2002:731-744.

72. Rosol TJ, Nagode LA, Couto CG, Hammer AS, Chew DJ, Peterson JC, Ayle RD, Steinmeyer CL, Capen CC. Parathyroid hormone (PTH)-related protein, PTH, and 1,25 dihydroxyvitamin A in dogs with cancer-associated hypercalcemia. Endocrinology 1992;31:1157-1164.

73. Klausner JS, Bell FW, Hayden DW, Hegstad RL, Johnston SD. Hypercalcemia in two cats with squamous cell carcinomas. J Am Vet Med Assoc 1990;196:103-105.

74. Sheafor SE, Gamblin RM, Couto CG. Hypercalcemia in two cats with multiple myeloma. J Am Anim Hosp Assoc 1996;32:503-508.

75. Rothenberg ME. Eosinophilia. N Engl J Med 1998;338:1592-1600.

76. Couto GC. Tumor associated eosinophilia in a dog. J Am Vet Med Assoc 1984;184:837-838.

77. Sellon RK, Rottman JB, Jordan HL, et al. Hypereosinophilia associated with transitional cell carcinoma in a cat. J Am Vet Med Assoc. 201: 591-593, 1992.

78. Huibregtse BA, Turner JL. Hypereosinophilic syndrome and eosinophilic leukemia: a comparison of 22 hypereosinophilic cats. J Am Anim Hosp Assoc 1994;30:591-599.

79. Plotnick A. Hypereosinophilic syndrome in a cat. Feline Pract 1994;22:27-31.

80. Byrne KP. Metabolic epidermal necrosis-hepatocutaneous syndrome. Vet Clin North Am 1999;29:1337-1355.

81. Ashley PF, Bowman LA. Symmetric cutaneous necrosis of the hind feet and multicentric follicular lymphoma in a cat. J Am Vet Med Assoc 1999;214:211-214.

82. Owen LN. TNM classification of tumors of domestic animals. 1st ed. Geneva, Switzerland: World Health Organization; 1980:46-47.

83. Moore AS, Cotter SM, Frimberger AE, et al. A comparison of doxorubicin and COP for maintenance of remission in cats with lymphosarcoma. J Vet Int Med 1996;10:372-375.

84. Madewell BR. Canine lymphosarcoma. Vet Clin North Am: Small Anim Pract. 1985;15:709-722.

85. Weller RE. Canine lymphosarcoma: current and future considerations. Proceedings of the Annual Kal Kan Symposium 1986;10:75-78.

86. Carter RF, Valli VEO. Advances in the cytologic diagnosis of canine lymphosarcoma. Semin Vet Med/Surg (Sm Anim). 1988;3:167-175.

87. Rosenthal RC, MacEwen EG. Treatment of lymphosarcoma in dogs. J Am Vet Med Assoc. 1990;196:774-781.

88. Rosenthal RC. The treatment of multicentric canine lymphosarcoma. Vet Clin North Am: Small Anim Pract. 1990;20:1093-1104.

89. Lieberman PH, Filippa DA, Straus DJ, Thaler HT, Cirrincione C, Clarkson BD. Evaluation of malignant lymphosarcomas using three classifications and the working formulation. Am J Med. 1986; 81:365-380.

90. Weller RE, Theilen GH, Madewell BR. Chemotherapeutic responses in dogs with lymphosarcoma and hypercalcemia. J Am Vet Med Assoc. 1982;181:891-893.

91. Valli VEO, McSherry BJ, Dunham BM, Jacobs RM, Lumsden JH. Histocytology of lymphoid tumors in the dog, cat and cow. Vet Pathol. 1981;18:494-512.

92. Cotter SM. Treatment of lymphosarcoma and leukemia with cyclophosphamide, vincristine and prednisone: I. Treatment of dogs. J Am Anim Hosp Assoc. 1983;19:159-165.

93. Rosenberg MP, Matus RE, PatnaikAK. Prognostic factors in dogs with lymphosarcoma and associated hypercalcemia. J Vet Int Med 1991; 5:268-271.

94. Mooney SC, Hayes AA, MacEwen EG, et al. Treatment and prognostic factors in lymphosarcoma in cats: 103 cases (1977-1981). J Amer Vet Med Assoc 1989; 194:696-702.

95. Rosenthal RC. Lymphosarcoma in dogs: chemotherapy. In: The Veterinary Clinics of North America, Small Animal Practice-Controversies in Clinical Oncology. Rosenthal RC and Jeglum KA, eds. WB Saunders Company, Philadelphia; 1996:26:1:63-71.

96. Price G, Page R, Fischer B, et al. Efficacy and toxocity of doxorubicin/cyclophosphamide maintenance therapy in dogs with multicentric lymphosarcoma. J Vet Intern Med 1991:5;259-262.

97. Hahn KA, Richardson RC, Teclaw RF, et al. Is maintenance chemotherapy appropriate for the management of canine malignant lymphosarcoma? J Vet Intern Med. 1992;6:3-10.

98. Vonderhaar MA. Evaluation of dogs with malignant lymphosarcoma treated with doxorubicin or epirubicin as single agent therapy. (Dissertation). West Lafayette, Indiana: Purdue University, 1994.

99. Carter RF, Harris CK, Withrow SJ, Valli VEO, Susaneck SJ. Chemotherapy of canine lymphosarcoma with histopathological correlation: Doxorubicin alone compared to COP as first treatment regimen. J Am Anim Hosp Assoc. 1987;23:587-596.

100. Vonderhaar MA, Morrison WB, DeNicola DB, et al. Comparison of duration of first remission using doxorubicin HCl versus epirubicin as single agent therapy for canine multicentric malignant lymphosarcoma. Proceedings of the Veterinary Cancer Society (abstract)1991;11: 87.

101. Vonderhaar MA, Morrison WB, Richardson RC, et al. Remission lengths of dogs with lymphosarcoma initially treated with doxorubicin HCl therapy. Proceedings of the American College of Veterinary Internal Medicine (abstract)1991;11:897.

102. Casazza AM, DiMarco A, Bertazzoli C, Formelli F, Giuliani F, Pratesi G. Antitumor activity, toxicity, and pharmacological properties of 4'-epiadriamycin. In: Siegenthaler W, Luthy R, eds. Current Chemotherapy: Proceedings of the Annual International Congress of Chemotherapy. 1978;10:1257-1260.

103. Cersosimo RJ, Hong WK. Epirubicin: a review of the pharmacology, clinical activity, and adverse effects of an adriamycin analogue. J Clin Oncol. 1986;4:425-439.

104. Ganzina F. 4'-epi-doxorubicin, a new analogue of doxorubicin: a preliminary overview of preclinical and clinical data. Cancer Treat Rep. 1983;10:1-22.

105. Vonderhaar MA, Morrison WB, Glickman NW, et al. Cardiac effects of doxorubicin and epirubicin as single agent therapy for canine malignant lymphosarcoma. Veterinary Cancer Society 14th Annual Conference Proceedings (abstract) 1994;29-30.

106. Vonderhaar MA, Morrison WB, Glickman NW, et al. Comparison of efficacy doxorubicin and epirubicin as single agent therapy for canine multicentric malignant lymphosarcoma. Veterinary Cancer Society 13th Annual Conference Proceedings (abstract) 1993; 46-47.

107. Moore AS, Ogilvie GK, Ruslander D, et al. Evaluation of mitoxantrone for the treatment of lymphosarcoma in dogs. J Amer Vet Med Assoc 1994:205; 1903-1905.

107a. Paeston AE, Maddison JE. Efficacy of doxorubicin as an induction agent for cats with lyphosarcoma. Aust Vet J 1999;77:442-444.

107b. Krista O, Lana SE, Ogilvie GK, Rand SW, Cotter SM, Moore AS. Single agent chemotherapy with doxorubicin for feline lymphoma: a retrospective study of 19 cases (1994-1997). J Vet Int Med 2001;15:125-130.

108. Moore AS. Treatment of feline lymphoma. Feline Pract 1996;24:17-20.

109. Moore A, Ruslander D, Rand W, et al. Toxicity and efficacy of oral idarubicin administration to cats with neoplasia. J Amer Vet Med Assoc 1995; 206:1550-1554.

110. Ogilvie G, Moore A, Obradovich J, et al. Toxicosis and efficacy associated with the administration of mitoxantrone to cats with malignant tumors. J Amer Vet Med Assoc 1993; 202:1839-1844.

111. MacEwen E, Hayes A, Matus R, et al. Evaluation of some prognostic factors for advanced multicentric lymphosarcoma in the dog: 147 cases (1978-1981). J Am Vet Med Assoc 1987:190; 564-568.

112. Stone MS, Goldstein MA, Cotter SM. Comparison of two protocols for induction of remission in dogs with lymphosarcoma. J Am Anim Hosp Assoc. 1991;27:315-321.

112a. Kitchell BE. Personal communication.

113. Keller E, MacEwen E, Rosenthal R, et al. Evaluation of prognostic factors and sequential combination chemotherapy for canine lymphosarcoma. J Vet Intern Med 1993:7; 289-295.

114. MacEwen EG, Rosenthal, Fox LE, et al. Evaluation of L-elsparaginase:polyethylene glycol conjugate versus native L-asparaginase combined with chemotherapy. A randomized double-blind study in canine lymphosarcoma. J Vet Int Med 1992:6; 230-234.

115. Matus RE. Chemotherapy of lymphosarcoma and leukemia. In: Current Veterinary Therapy X. Small Animal Practice. Kirk RW (ed), WB Saunders Co, Philadelphia, 1989:482-488.

116. Cotter SM. Treatment of lymphosarcoma and leukemia with cyclophosphamide, vincristine and prednisone: II. Treatment of cats. J Amer Anim Hosp Assoc 1983; 19:166-172.

117. Jeglum KA, Whereat A, Young K. Chemotherapy of lymphosarcoma in 75 cats. J Amer Vet Med Assoc 1987; 190:174-178.

118. Mauldin GE, Mooney SC, Meleo KA, et al. Chemotherapy in 132 cats with lymphosarcoma: 1988-1994.Veterinary Cancer Society 14th Annual Conference Proceedings. 1995; Abstract. p.35-36.

119. O'Keefe DA, Sisson DD, Gelberg HB, et al. Systemic toxicity associated with doxorubicin administration in cats. J Vet Intern Med 1993;7:309-317.

120. Morrison WB. Principles of treating chemotherapy complications. In: Morrison WB (ed). Cancer in Dogs and Cats: Medical and Surgical Management. 2nd ed. Jackson, WY: Teton NewMedia 2002:365-374.

121. Decorti G, Klugmann FB, Candussio L, Furlani A, Scarcia V, Baldini L. Uptake of adriamycin by rat and mouse mast cells and correlation with histamine release. Cancer Res 1989;49;1921-1926.

122. Bristow MR, Sageman WS, Scott RH, Bellingham ME, Bowden RE, Kernoff RS, Snidow GH, Daniels JR. Acute and chronic cardiovascular effects of doxorubicin in the dog: the cardiovascular pharmacology of drug-induced histamine release. J Cardiovasc Pharmacol 1980;2:487-515.

123. Van Vleet JF, Ferrans VJ. Clinical observations, cutaneous lesions, and hematologic alterations in chronic adriamycin intoxication in dogs with and without vitamin E and selenium supplementation. Am J Vet Res 1980;41:691-699.

124. Richardson RC, Hahn K, Knapp D, Bonney P, Hahn L, Morrison WB. Hematologic changes associated with epirubicin and doxorubicin during the first 21 days following administration. Proceedings of the Veterinary Cancer Society Conference (abstract)1988;8:22.

125. O'Keef DA, Schaeffer DJ. Hematologic toxicosis associated with doxorubicin administration in cats. J Vet Int Med 1992;6:276-282.

126. Badylak SF, Van Vleet JF, Herman EH, Ferrans VJ, Meyers CE. Pokilocytosis in dogs with chronic doxorubicin toxicosis. Am J Vet Res 1985;46:505-508.

127. Pond EC, Morrow EC. Hepatotoxicity associated with methotrexate therapy in a dog. J Small Anim Pract 1982;23:659-666.

128. Ogilvie GK, Richardson RC, Curtis CR, Withrow SJ, Reynolds HA, Norris AM, Henderson RA, Klausner JS, Fowler JD, McCaw D. Acute and short-term toxicoses associated with the administration of doxorubicin to dogs with malignant tumors, J Am Vet Med Assoc 1989;195:1584-1587.

129. Morrison WB, Vonderhaar MA, Hamilton TA, Hahn L. Pancreatitis associated with cytotoxic drug therapy for malignant neoplasia in dogs. Proceedings of the Veterinary Cancer Society (abstract) 1991;11:73.

130. Vonderhaar MA, Morrison WB, Glickman NW, Varshovsky JA, DeNicola DB, Carlton WC, Richardson RC. Comparison of efficacy of doxorubicin and epirubicin as single agent therapy for canine multicentric malignant lymphoma. Proceedings of the Veterinary Cancer Society (abstract)1994;13:46.

131. Chabner BA, Myers CE. Antitumor antibiotics. In: DeVita VT, Hellman S, Rosenberg SA. Cancer: Principles and Practice of Oncology. 4th ed. Philadelphia: J B Lippincott Co 1993.

132. Loar AS, Susaneck SJ. Doxorubicin-induced cardiotoxicity in five dogs. Sem Vet Med Surg (Small Animal) 1986;1:68-71.

133. Susaneck SJ. Doxorubicin therapy in the dog. J Am Vet Med Assoc 1983;182:70-72.

134. Knapp DW, Richardson RC, DeNicola DB, Long GG, Blevins WE. Cisplatin toxicity in cats. J Vet Int Med 1987;1:29-35.

135. Shen AS, Haslett C, Feldsien DC, Henson PM, Cherniack RM. The intensity of chronic lung inflammation and fibrosis after bleomycin is directly related to the severity of acute injury. Am Rev Respir Dis 1988;137:564-571.

136. Charney SC, Bergman PJ, Hohenhaus AE, McKnight JA. Risk factors for sterile hemorrhagic cystitis in dogs with lymphoma receiving cyclophosphamide with or without concurrent administration of furosemide: 216 cases (1990-1996). J Am Vet Med Assoc 2003;222:1288-1393.

137. Peterson JL, Couto CG, Hammer AS, Ayl RD. Acute sterile hemorrhagic cystitis after a single intravenous administration of cyclophosphamide in three dogs. J Am Vet Med Assoc 1992;201:1572-1574.

138. L 'Heureux D. Hemorrhagic cystitis: a unique toxicity. Veterinary Cancer Society Newsletter 1996;20:11.

139. Page R. Cisplatin, a new antineoplastic drug in veterinary medicine. J Am Vet Med Assoc 1985;186:288-290.

140. Daugaard G, Rossing N, RΔrth M. Effects of cisplatin on the different measures of glomerular function in the human kidney with special emphasis on high-dose. Cancer Chemother Pharmacol 1988;21:163-167.

141. Hamilton TA, Cook JR, Braund KG, Morrison WB, Mehta JR. Vincristine-induced peripheral neuropathy in a dog. J AM Vet Med Assoc 1991;198:635-638.

142. Benitah N, De Lorimier L, Gaspar M, Kitchell BE. Chlorambucil-induced myoclonus in a cat with lymphoma. J Am Anim Hosp Assoc 2003;39:283-287.

143. Meleo KA. The role of radiotherapy in the treatment of lymphoma and thymoma. Vet Clinics North Am 1997;27:115-129.

144. Laing EG, Fritzpatrick PJ, Binnington AG, et al: Half-body radiotherapy in the treatment of canine lymphoma. J Vet Int Med 1989;3:102-108.

145. Giger U, Evans SM, Hendrick MJ, Dudek SM. Orthovoltage radiotherapy of primary lymphoma of bone in a dog. J Am Vet Med Assoc 1989;195:627-630.

146. Gustafson NR, LaRue SM. Radiation therapy as an adjuvant to chemotherapy for the treatment of canine lymphoma: an update on toxicities and remission times. Veterinary Cancer Society Proceedings (abstract) 2002;22:28.

147. Madewell BR. Diagnosis, assessment of prognosis, and treatment of dogs with lymphoma: the sentinal changes (1973-1999). J Vet Int Med 1999;13:393-394.

148. Elmslie RE, Ogilvie GK, Gillette EL, McChesney-Gillette S. Radiotherapy with and without chemotherapy for localized lymphoma in 10 cats. Vet Rad 1991;32:277-280.

149. Williams L. Unpublished data.

150. Ogilvie GK. Alterations in metabolism and nutritional support for veterinary cancer patients: recent advances. Comp Cont Ed 1993;7:925-936.

151. Morrison WB, Roth JA, Goff BL, Stewart-Brown B, Incefy GS, Arp LA. Orally administered clonidine as a secretagogue of growth hormone and as a thymotrophic agent in dogs of various ages. Am J Vet Res 1990;51:65-70.

152. Ogilvie GK, FettmanMJ, Mallinckrodt CH, Walton JA, Hansen RA, Davenport DJ, Gross KL, Richardson KS, Rogers Q, Hand MS. Effect of fish oil, arginine, and doxorubicin chemotherapy on remission and survival time for dogs with lymphoma. Cancer 2000;88:1916-1928.

153. Morrison WB. Unpublished data.

154. Vonderhaar MA. Evaluation of dogs with malignant lymphosarcoma treated with doxorubicin or epirubicin as single agent therapy. (Thesis). West Lafayette, Indiana: Purdue University, 1994.

155. Van Vechten M, Helfand SC, Jeglum KA. Treatment of relapsed canine lymphoma with doxorubicin and dacarbazine. J Vet Int Med 1990;4:187-191.

156. Lucroy MD, Phillips BS, Kraegel SA, Simonson ER, Madewell BR. Evaluation of single-agent mitoxantrone as chemotherapy for relapsing canine lymphoma. J Vet Intern Med 1998;12:325-329.

157. Hammer AS, Couto CG, Ayle RD, Shank KA. Treatment of tumor-bearing dogs with actinomycin D. J Vet Intern Med 1994;8:236-239.

158. Moore AS, Ogilvie GL, Vail DM. Actinomycin D for re-induction of remission in dogs with resistant lymphoma. J Vet Intern Med 1994;8:343-344.

159. Moore AS, London CA, Wood CA, Williams LE, Cotter SM, L'Heureux DA, Frimberger AE. Lomustine (CCNU) for the treatment of resistant lymphoma in dogs. J Vet Intern Med 1999;13:395-398.

160. Paoloni MC, Helfand SC, Burgess KE, Poirier VJ, Turek MM, Kurzman ID, Vail DM. Lomustine as a rescue agent for canine lymphoma: efficacy and safety profile. Mid-Year Proceedings of the Veterinary Cancer Society (abstract).2002:12.

161. Wiedemann AL, Jones PD, deLorimier LP, Fan TM, Kitchell BE. Use of lomustine (CCNU) as a monotherapeutic rescue agent in relapsed canine lymphoma previously treated with COPLA. Mid-Year Proceedings of the Veterinary Cancer Society (abstract), 2002:22.

162. Helfand SC. Personal communication. Goldschmidt MH. Cutaneous lymphosarcoma. In: Skin Tumors of the Dog and Cat. Goldschmidt MH and Shofer FS, (eds). Pergamon Press Oxford pp.252-264.

163. Couto CG. Cutaneous lymphosarcomas. Proceedings of the 11th Kal Kan Symposium 1987; 71-77.

164. Caciolo PL, Nesbitt GH, Patnaik AK, Hayes AA. Cutaneous lymphosarcoma in the cat: a report of nine cases. J Am Anim Hosp Assoc 1984; 20: 491-496.

165. Beale KM, Bolon B. Canine cutaneous lymphosarcoma: epitheliotropic and non-epitheliotropic, a retrospective study. In: Advances in Veterinary Dermatology, Ihrke. PJ, Mason IS and White SD, eds. Vol 2 : 1992 Pergamon Press, Oxford pp.273-284.

166. Souza CHM, Valli VE, Kitchell BE, Evandro T-P. Immunohistochemical detection of retinoid receptors in cutaneous lymphoma in dogs. Mid-Year Proceedings of the Veterinary Cancer Society (abstract), 2002:20.

167. Brown NO, Nesbitt GH, Patnaik AK, MacEwen EG. Cutaneous lymphosarcoma in the dog: a disease with variable clinical and histologic manifestations. J Am Anim Hosp Assoc 1980;16:565-572.

168. Plant JD. Would you have diagnosed cutaneous epitheliotropic lymphosarcoma in these two cats? Vet Med 1991; Augus:801-806.

169. Caciolo PL, Hayes AA, Patnaik AK, et al. A case of mycosis fungoides in a cat and literature review. J Am Anim Hosp Assoc 1983; 19:505-512.

170. Lemarie SL, Eddlestone SM. Treatment of cutaneous T-cell lymphosarcoma with dacarbazine in a dog. Vet Derm 1997: 8:41-46.

171. Moore PF, Olivery T. Cutaneous lymphosarcomas in companion animals. Clin Derm 1994; 499-505.

172. White SD, Rosychuk RA, Scott KV, et al. Use of isotretinoin and etretinate for the treatment of benign cutaneous neoplasia and cutaneous lymphosarcoma in dogs. J Amer Vet Med Assoc 1993; 202:387-391.

173. Beale KM, Dill-Mackey E, Meyer DJ, Calderwood-Mays M. An unusual presentation of cutaneous lymphosarcoma in two dogs. J Am Anim Hosp Assoc 1990; 26:429-432.

174. Baker JL, Scott DW. Mycosis fungoides in two cats. J Am Anim Hosp Assoc 1989 25:97-101.

175. DeBoer DJ, Turrel JM, Moore PF. Mycosis fungoides in a dog: demonstration of T-cell specificity and response to radiotherapy. J Am Anim Hosp Assoc 1990; 26:566-572.

176. Power HT, Ihrke PJ. Retinoids in veterinary dermatology. Vet Clin North Am Small Anim Prac 1990; 20:1525-1539.

177. Kwochka KW. Retinoids in veterinary dermatology. In: Kirk RW, ed. Current Veterinary Therapy X. Philadelphia: WB Saunders Co, 1989: 553-560.

Index

Page numbers followed by an *f* indicate a figure; page numbers followed by a *t* indicate a table.

Printed and bound by CPI Group (UK) Ltd, Croydon, CR0 4YY

23/10/2024

01777696-0008